More Advance Praise for
Neuroimmunology

"Autoimmune disorders are assuming ...ıe diagnosis and management of neurological dis , using a case report format, succinctly and clearly presents tı . recent knowledge on the diagnostic approach to and the best treatment of the entire spectrum of autoimmune disorders that affect the nervous system. The book can be profitably read both by general physicians and experienced neurologists. It can serve either as a reference to answer a question on a specific disorder or read from cover to cover to achieve a broad overview of the subject. I did the latter; it was both informative and entertaining."
 —*Jerome B. Posner, MD, Evelyn Frew American Cancer Society Clinical Research Professor, Memorial Sloan-Kettering Cancer Center, New York, NY*

"Recognition of immune-mediated central and peripheral nerve system disorders is increasing. The collection of neuroimmunological disorders by Aaron Miller and Tracy DeAngelis is comprehensive. Each case includes a valuable differential diagnosis, practical discussion of management, and update of the latest on pathogenesis of disease. Neurology residents, neurologists preparing for board examinations, as well as active clinical neurologists will frequently take this volume from their bookshelves to help guide their diagnosis and treatment. The authors are to be congratulated for a fine addition to the neurologic literature."
 —*Don Gilden, MD, Louise Baum Endowed Chair and Professor, Department of Neurology, University of Colorado School of Medicine, Aurora, CO*

OXFORD
UNIVERSITY PRESS

Oxford University Press, Inc., publishes works that further Oxford University's objective of excellence
in research, scholarship, and education.

Oxford New York
Auckland Cape Town Dar es Salaam Hong Kong Karachi
Kuala Lumpur Madrid Melbourne Mexico City Nairobi
New Delhi Shanghai Taipei Toronto

With offices in
Argentina Austria Brazil Chile Czech Republic France Greece
Guatemala Hungary Italy Japan Poland Portugal Singapore
South Korea Switzerland Thailand Turkey Ukraine Vietnam

Copyright © 2012 by Oxford University Press, Inc.

Published by Oxford University Press, Inc.
198 Madison Avenue, New York, New York 10016
www.oup.com

First issued as an Oxford University Press paperback, 2012

Oxford is a registered trademark of Oxford University Press

Library of Congress Cataloging-in-Publication Data
Miller, Aaron E.
Neuroimmunology / Aaron E. Miller, Teresa M. DeAngelis.
     p. ; cm.—(What do I do now?)
  Includes bibliographical references and index.
  ISBN 978-0-19-973292-0 (pbk.)
  I. DeAngelis, Teresa M. II. Title. III. Series: What do I do now?.
  [DNLM: 1. Autoimmune Diseases of the Nervous System—diagnosis—Case
Reports. 2. Autoimmune Diseases of the Nervous System—therapy—Case
Reports. 3. Nervous System—immunology—Case Reports. WL 141]
LC classification not assigned
616.97'8—dc23   2011030225

Printed in the United States of America on acid-free paper

This book is dedicated to:

Ellen, who has made my professional career possible and the rest of my life wonderful.

—AEM

My dear Luke and Sunny, who grew in parallel with this book. And always, to Captain Billy.

—TMD

Preface

Patients with various types of neuroimmunological disorders are seen in both the office and on the wards. Navigating even commonly encountered conditions such as multiple sclerosis or myasthenia gravis can make some neurologists feel like they are out of their comfort zone. Identifying and managing more rare syndromes such as autoimmune paraneoplastic encephalitidies can prompt the clinician to ask, "What do I do now?"

In the neuroimmunology handbook of the "What Do I Do Now?" series, our goal was to provide a useful framework for clinicians to employ when approaching challenging immune-mediated diseases of both the central and peripheral nervous systems. Each chapter includes a case presentation followed by a discussion focusing on localization, differential diagnosis and the critical aspects of both diagnostic evaluation and treatment specific to the case and disorder itself. We aimed to present a range of conditions, from commonly encountered disorders such as demyelinating disease, to more rare presentations like Hashimoto's encephalopathy. Our recommendations for diagnostic testing and therapeutic approaches rest, whenever possible, on available current evidence. Key clinical points are highlighted at the conclusion of each chapter, along with a list of important references. In select chapters, tables and figures are provided to illustrate cardinal teaching points such as diagnostic criterion.

We crafted this volume to be an accessible tool for neurologists and clinicians at all levels of training. Our hope is that it will be an important and useful resource for both clinicians and their patients in helping to facilitate better recognition and management of neuroimmunological disorders and improve patient care.

Tracy M. DeAngelis, MD
Aaron E. Miller, MD

Acknowledgments

Many of the cases described in this book involve challenging presentations of neuroimmunological disorders requiring the expertise and support of a multidisciplinary clinical care team. In addition to our colleagues from neurology, we acknowledge the invaluable collaboration with our colleagues in the fields of neuroradiology, neuro-ophthalmology, rheumatology, internal medicine, critical care neuro-intensivists, among others. In addition, we would like to recognize the residents and fellows at the front lines of managing such difficult cases at Mount Sinai and everywhere, for their diligence, commitment and dedication to patient care that inspires us daily. We would also like to extend our sincerest gratitude to the team at Oxford University Press, Craig Panner and Kathryn Winder, for their help, support and persistence in bringing this volume to completion.

Tracy M. DeAngelis, MD
Aaron E. Miller, MD

Contents

2 Acute Disseminated Encephalomyelitis

A 25-year-old male college student is brought to his primary care physician with complaints of two days of double vision, tingling involving his right foot, unsteady gait, and mild confusion. He is otherwise healthy without any past medical history apart from an episode of infectious mononucleosis at age 15. He is seen by his primary care physician, who finds him to be encephalopathic with a dystaxic gait and refers him to the local emergency room for urgent evaluation. On neurologic examination, he is oriented to self and place but does not know the date, and his mentation is slow. Extraocular movements reveal left internuclear ophthalmoplegia with right abducting nystagmus and a left adduction palsy. Sensory examination is significant for diminished vibration and joint position sense involving his right foot. His motor strength demonstrates full power with diffuse hyperreflexia and a right extensor plantar response. Gait is moderately dystaxic with a steppage quality to the right lower extremity. He denies any headache, fever, recent infections, or travel. He takes no medications but reports receiving the seasonal flu vaccination two weeks prior to the onset of symptoms. The patient is admitted for further evaluation, and MRIs of the brain and spine with and without contrast are performed, which demonstrate multiple T2/FLAIR hyperintense periventricular and subcortical white matter lesions, the majority of which demonstrate gadolinium enhancement, some with a distinct open-ring enhancement pattern (Fig. 2-1). A lesion in the left rostral midbrain demonstrates enhancement. MRIs of the cervical and thoracic spine demonstrate three intramedullary lesions, two of which enhance. A lumbar puncture is performed, which discloses a lymphocytic pleocytosis with 26 cells, elevated protein of 55, negative HSV-2 PCR, Lyme serology, VDRL, and normal cytology. IgG synthesis and index are elevated and cerebrospinal fluid (CSF) oligoclonal bands are absent.

What do you do now?

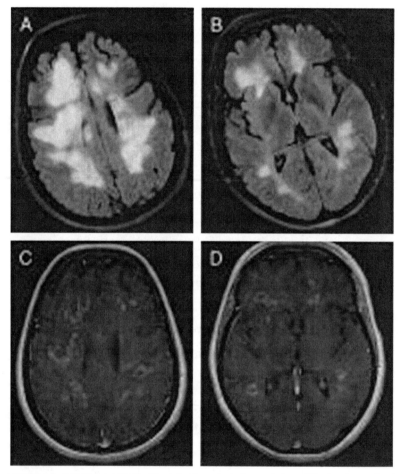

FIGURE 2-1 MRI from a patient with acute disseminated encephalomyelitis showing contrast enhancement in nearly all lesions (lower panels). The upper panels show the lesions hyperintense on T2-weighted imaging. (Reprinted with permission from Bermel RA, Fox RJ. MRI in multiple sclerosis. *Continuum: Lifelong Learning in Neurology* 2010; 16(5):46.)

This patient presents with a post-vaccinal neurologic syndrome with multifocal symptomatology and deficits with supratentorial and infratentorial involvement, as well as encephalopathy. MR imaging demonstrates multiple T2/FLAIR hyperintense white matter abnormalities involving both the brain and spinal cord, the majority of which demonstrate gadolinium enhancement, including an open-ring enhancement pattern radiographically characteristic of demyelination. This presentation is highly suspicious for acute disseminated encephalomyelitis (ADEM), a typically monophasic syndrome that occurs often in close temporal association to an immunization or systemic viral infection, the latter either a post- or parainfectious process. Children are preferentially affected. Recurrent, relapsing, and multiphasic forms of ADEM have been described in the literature; however, these presentations remain controversial and poorly defined. Various vaccines and systemic infections have been linked to ADEM, including influenza, varicella zoster, herpes simplex, measles, mumps, rubella, *Borrelia burgdorfei*, mycoplasma, and Epstein-Barr virus. Of note, however, ADEM, more often than not, develops in the absence of any antecedent infection.

The onset of ADEM is generally rapid and peak neurologic dysfunction manifests within several days. Clinical symptoms are multifocal and varied, including encephalopathy, cerebral hemispheric deficits such as hemiparesis and hemisensory loss, brain stem dysfunction, myelopathy, as well as seizures. The degree of encephalopathy can range from mild lethargy and confusion to frank coma. Rarely, a hyperacute, severe variant of ADEM occurs, referred to as acute hemorrhagic leukoencephalitis (AHLE), which pathologically involves petechial hemorrhage and venular necrosis. In cases of AHLE, CSF analysis generally demonstrates increased opening pressure, elevated protein, and a pleocytosis of both red and white blood cells. As such, the differential diagnosis here would include hemorrhagic, necrotizing infectious processes such as herpes simplex meningoencephalitis, brain abscesses, and neoplasms such as metastatic melanoma. Cases similar to neuromyelitis optica with bilateral optic neuropathy and longitudinally extensive spinal cords lesions have also been described, often in the pediatric population. Peripheral nervous system involvement has been described, in the form of acute polyradiculoneuropathies, more commonly in adult rather than pediatric presentations.

ADEM can be difficult to distinguish from a severe, fulminant first episode of multiple sclerosis (MS), but differentiating these two entities has critical long-term therapeutic implications. ADEM is typically a self-limited illness and does not require the chronic immunomodulatory or immunosuppressive therapeutics of MS. Various differentiating factors and diagnostic criteria have been proposed for ADEM, with considerable degrees of controversy regarding their reliability. Factors suggested as supportive of ADEM include the presence of encephalopathy, seizures, radiographic presence of poorly marginated, large, sometimes tumefactive-sized lesions, deep gray matter and cortical lesions, and a predominance of gadolinium-enhancing lesions. Both incomplete and complete ring-shaped patterns of enhancement had been described. Meningeal enhancement is considered unusual. Lesions on MRI in ADEM tend to at least partially resolve, although sometimes they can persist on serial imaging, which is more characteristic of demyelinating plaques in MS. The absence of CSF oligoclonal bands (OCBs), commonly identified in MS patients, is considered to favor ADEM, but the utility of OCB positivity remains unknown, as 58% and 29% of adult and pediatric ADEM cases, respectively, have OCBs. In cases with significant clinical and paraclinical overlap, the judgment of whether to initiate immunomodulatory therapy can be difficult, and most patients are followed with close clinical and radiographic surveillance to ascertain new evidence of disease activity over the subsequent months. In addition to demyelinating disease, other candidate differential diagnoses for ADEM include cerebral vasculitis, multiple infarcts, chronic meningitides, neoplastic processes, and granulomatous disease. Brain biopsy is sometimes required to differentiate these alternative entities form ADEM.

Treatment of ADEM generally involves high-dose intravenous methylprednisolone, sometimes followed by oral steroid tapering doses, as well as immunotherapies such as plasma exchange or intravenous immunoglobulin in corticosteroid-refractory cases. Close respiratory monitoring in an intensive care unit is often recommended because of the possibility of respiratory compromise secondary to brain stem involvement and severe encephalopathy. The prognosis with therapy, however, is uniformly reported as favorable, but recovery time can vary from weeks to months.

- ADEM, an immune-mediated, inflammatory, demyelinating disorder of the central nervous system, is a post-infectious or post-vaccinal classically monophasic illness, although controversial multiphasic and relapsing forms have been described.
- There is a wide variability in the severity of ADEM presentations, but in the majority of cases it is a self-limited illness with a favorable prognosis.
- ADEM can be difficult to distinguish from a fulminant, initial episode of MS, necessitating ongoing close clinical and radiographic surveillance for new disease activity suggestive of the latter.

Further Reading

DeSeze J, Debouverie M, Zephir H, et al. Acute fulminant demyelinating disease: a descriptive study of 60 patients. *Arch Neurol* 2007; 64:1426-1432.

Krupp LB, Banwell B, Tenembaum S. International Pediatric MS Study Group. Consensus definitions proposed for pediatric multiple sclerosis and related disorders. *Neurology* 2007; 68(16 Suppl 2):S7-S12.

Young NP, Weinshenker BG, Lucchinetti CF. Acute disseminated encephalomyelitis: current understanding and controversies. *Semin Neurol* 2008; 28:84-94.

3 Optic Neuritis

A 36-year-old white woman noted blurred vision in her left eye when she tried to apply makeup in the morning before going to work. She also experienced pain on eye movement. She denies any other recent symptoms. Her past medical history is positive for migraine headaches that have occurred approximately every two months since she was an adolescent. The headaches are characterized as unilateral throbbing pain, accompanied by photo- and phonophobia and scintillating scotomata, but they are "very different" from the blurred vision she is currently experiencing. She also has a history of irritable bowel syndrome and depression, for which she currently takes escitalopram. She describes her recent mood as "fine." Her other medications are diazepam and famotidine. She works as an office manager and lives with her husband, two healthy children, and a pet cat. She does not smoke and seldom drinks alcohol.

On physical examination, the patient is a well-developed well-nourished woman with BP 110/60, pulse 70 and regular, and respiratory rate of 12. Temporal pulses are normal and no carotid bruits are present.

Inspection of the eyes is normal. Mental status is normal. Visual acuity is 20/200 in the left eye, 20/20 in the right eye. She reports color desaturation in the left eye when she is presented with a red object. A relative afferent pupillary defect is noted in the left eye. Funduscopy reveals no abnormalities, including normal-appearing optic discs bilaterally (Figs. 3.1-3.3). The remainder of the neurologic examination is entirely normal.

What do you do now?

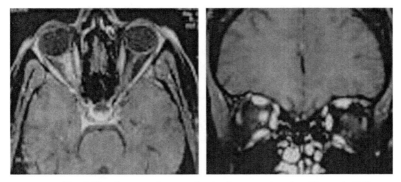

FIGURE 3-1 The right optic nerve shows contrast enhancement and swelling on both the axial (left) and coronal (right) views. (Reprinted with permission from Costello F. Retrobulbar optic neuropathies. *Continuum: Lifelong Learning in Neurology* 2009; 15(4):49.)

4   Transverse Myelitis

You are asked to evaluate a 39-year-old woman, previously entirely healthy, who had awakened the previous day with a feeling of pressure in the chest. When she lay down she found that her entire left side was weak and her right side somewhat less so. After arrival at the hospital, the emergency department staff decided that she "did not have a stroke" and admitted her for further evaluation. Over the next 24 hours her condition worsened and she reported that she could not move either leg or her left arm. She stated that her legs felt as if she had received an epidural anesthetic. Since admission to the hospital she has been unable to urinate. On examination, the patient is awake and alert with normal cranial nerve function. She has no movement in either leg or the left arm and mild weakness in the entire right arm. She cannot feel pinprick below the breast and the sensation is reduced to a level of C6 bilaterally. Joint position sense is markedly impaired in all extremities. Vibration sense is absent in the legs and reduced in the

fingers bilaterally. Deep tendon reflexes are 1+
throughout and plantar responses are silent.

What do you do now?

This is a case of fulminant myelopathy. In such circumstances, one of your first obligations is to make certain that the clinical manifestations are not due to cord compression, which might require urgent surgical intervention. Thus, obtaining an MRI of the cervical spine is critical in such situations. Assuming cord compression is absent, you can then consider alternative diagnoses. In very acute cases of severe myelopathy, anterior spinal artery infarction is a possibility. However, the vascular territory of the anterior spinal artery spares the posterior columns, so the patient will generally not manifest impairment of joint position or vibratory sensation.

More likely etiologies of acute to subacute myelopathy include infectious or inflammatory causes. The former, which are relatively uncommon, are likely to be accompanied by other stigmata of the infection. For example, neuroborreliosis (Lyme disease) may cause a myelopathy, but there is usually history of the typical "bull's-eye" rash (erythema chronicum migrans), arthritis, and/or cardiac involvement. Varicella zoster virus may cause myelitis, but usually in the setting of cutaneous herpes zoster and particularly in immunocompromised individuals. Occasionally skin lesions are absent, in which case the diagnosis can be made by detecting VZV in cerebrospinal fluid (CSF) by polymerase chain reaction. Neurosyphilis is likely to be associated with a meningitic process, and diagnosis, as with other infections, will also be facilitated by CSF examination. In neurosyphilis, the diagnosis may be confirmed by finding a reactive serum treponemal antibody assay or a reactive CSF pleocytosis or reactive VDRL. Intramedullary spinal cord parasitic infections are quite uncommon in North America, but such entities as schistosomiasis or cysticercosis may be suspected in patients from parts of the world where these disorders are endemic.

Very often the differential diagnosis of acute to subacute myelopathy comes down to distinguishing among the entities of acute disseminated encephalomyelitis (ADEM), idiopathic transverse myelitis (ITM), an initial spinal cord presentation of multiple sclerosis (MS), and neuromyelitis optica (NMO) spectrum disorder. In most cases, you will be able to make at least a probable diagnosis after obtaining spinal and brain MRIs and, in some cases, performing a lumbar puncture.

ADEM, which is discussed in greater detail in Chapter 2, seldom presents as a pure myelopathy. It is much more likely to involve the brain, either alone or in combination with the spinal cord. Patients will frequently have alterations in mental status or seizures, as well as focal neurologic signs. Brain MRI will typically reveal large, fluffy, bilateral lesions that are hyperintense on T2-weighted sequences and all (or nearly all) enhance after administration of gadolinium.

Classical NMO (also known as Devic's disease) will be discussed more extensively in Chapter 5. However, as part of the NMO spectrum disorders, myelitis alone may occur. The hallmark of this condition, however, in distinction to the other inflammatory myelopathies, is the presence of a longitudinally extensive intramedullary spinal cord lesion, generally extending over at least three vertebral bodies. NMO spectrum disorders are associated with antibodies to aquaporin 4 water channels, and the NMO-Ig antibody test, directed against this antigen, has been reported to be positive in approximately a third to a half of patients with longitudinally extensive transverse myelitis.

The majority of patients presenting with acute to subacute myelopathy will prove to have either ITM or a myelopathic form of the so-called clinically isolated syndrome (CIS)—that is, the first clinical manifestation of what will ultimately prove to be MS. Some clinical features may help to distinguish between these two possibilities. In ITM, the myelopathy is more likely to be very severe, with marked, often symmetrical, motor weakness and usually a sensory level to pain and temperature. Spinal MRI is more likely to show a lesion involving most of the cord at the affected level, often causing cord swelling. The Transverse Myelitis Consortium Working Group has proposed diagnostic criteria for idiopathic acute transverse myelitis (Table 4-1). In contrast, when the myelopathy is an initial manifestation of MS, the clinical symptoms are often relatively mild, asymmetrical, and predominantly sensory. The cord lesion, as demonstrated on MRI, is more likely to be partial (usually occupying less than half the cord diameter), tending most often to be located posterolaterally. The most important distinguishing feature between ITM and myelopathic CIS, however, is the presence of T2 hyperintense lesions on brain MRI in the latter. When an inflammatory myelopathy is accompanied by at least two T2 hyperintensities, the probability of subsequent diagnosis of MS may exceed 90%, and such patients should be considered for treatment with disease-modifying therapies for MS (as further discussed in Chapter 3 on optic neuritis).

TABLE 4-1 **The Transverse Myelitis Consortium Working Group Proposed Diagnostic Criteria for Idiopathic Acute Transverse Myelitis**

- Bilateral (not necessarily symmetric) sensorimotor or autonomic spinal cord dysfunction
- Maximal worsening of clinical deficits between 4 hours and 21 days
- Evidence of spinal cord inflammation (either CSF pleocytosis or elevated IgG index or gadolinium-enhancing cord lesion)
- Exclusion of spinal cord compression

Patients with the typical syndrome of fulminant myelitis, accompanied by nearly complete involvement of the spinal cord segment, and the absence of brain MRI lesions have a very low probability (in the range of 10%) of ultimately developing a second clinical episode that would make the diagnosis of MS.

Some patients experience transverse myelitis as a manifestation of a systemic illness. Usually the underlying illness has other stigmata, but occasionally transverse myelitis will be the initial manifestation of such entities as systemic lupus erythematosus, sarcoidoisis, Sjögren's syndrome, or Behçet's disease. Investigation for these possibilities may be warranted even in the absence of other system involvement.

The CSF examination results in cases of ITM and CIS are not generally distinguishable, although the latter may be more likely to demonstrate the presence of oligoclonal bands and evidence of the quantitative increase in the production of immunoglobulin (e.g., increased IgG index). Both syndromes may exhibit mild to moderate mononuclear cell pleocytosis (usually fewer than 50 cells). Occasionally a much higher CSF cell count may be found in ITM. In the case of myelopathy as an NMO spectrum disorder, often a more prominent pleocytosis, frequently including neutrophils, is present and oligoclonal bands, although possible, occur much less often than with MS.

This patient demonstrated a nearly full-thickness T2 hyperintense lesion at the C4 level that longitudinally extended for only one segment. It enhanced after the administration of gadolinium. Brain MRI was normal. CSF demonstrated 27 mononuclear cells, normal glucose, and a protein of 60 mg/dL. Oligoclonal bands were not present and the IgG index was normal. Thus, this patient's diagnosis is most likely ITM.

You should treat this patient with a course of high-dose intravenous methylprednisolone (e.g., 1000 mg daily for 5 days). Although controlled randomized trials in ITM have not been conducted, it is likely that such treatment will hasten recovery. Patients who do not improve with steroids may be considered for treatment with plasmapheresis, which has been shown to offer a 43% chance of improvement (compared to 8% with sham pheresis) in patients with a variety of inflammatory/demyelinating conditions that have been refractory to IV corticosteroids.

The ultimate recovery from ITM is quite variable; in one series more than 75% were able to walk independently. This patient made an excellent recovery and was left with only very mild weakness and spasticity in the left leg. She has now been followed for nearly a decade with no further neurologic symptoms and a brain MRI that has remained normal.

KEY POINTS TO REMEMBER

- In a patient with a fulminant myelopathy, it is critical to rule out spinal cord compression.
- The most likely etiologies of acute to subacute myelopathy are infectious or inflammatory.
- When an inflammatory myelopathy is accompanied by the presence of at least two T2 hyperintensities, the probability of subsequent diagnosis of MS may exceed 90%, and such patients should be considered for treatment with disease-modifying therapies for MS.
- Patients with the typical syndrome of fulminant myelitis, accompanied by nearly complete involvement of the spinal cord segment, and the absence of brain MRI lesions have a very low probability (in the range of 10%) of ultimately developing a second clinical episode that would make the diagnosis of MS.

Further Reading

Frohman EM, Wingerchuk DM. Clinical practice. Transverse myelitis. *N Engl J Med* 2010; 363(6):564-572.

Sá MJ. Acute transverse myelitis: a practical reappraisal. *Autoimmun Rev* 2009; 9(2): 128-131.

Wingerchuk DM. Infectious and inflammatory myelopathies. *Continuum* 2008; 14(3):36-57.

5   Neuromyelitis Optica

A 52-year-old nurse previously given a diagnosis of multiple sclerosis (MS) presents for outpatient evaluation for treatment recommendations. Seventeen years ago, she presented with two episodes of myelitis involving paresthesias of her bilateral upper extremities and subsequently an attack of severe lower extremity weakness. Diagnostic evaluation included an MRI of the brain and spinal cord, which demonstrated two longitudinally extensively T2 hyperintense enhancing lesions spanning C2–C7 and T2–T6 levels (Fig. 5-1). MRI of the brain was unremarkable. CSF studies at the time revealed a moderate pleocytosis of 26 cells with neutrophilic predominance, elevated protein, and elevated IgG synthesis without oligoclonal bands. She was diagnosed with MS and treated with a course of high-dose IV corticosteroids with good recovery. She remained asymptomatic for the subsequent 7 years; however, thereafter, she began to experience frequent attacks, approximately every 3 months, of lower extremity weakness. With each episode, she received a course of high-dose IV corticosteroids, but with progressively limited recoveries after each episode. The following year she began using a cane, and by the next year she was wheelchair-bound due to a severe spastic paraparesis of the lower extremities. MRI spinal cord surveys continued to demonstrate spans of longitudinally extensive myelitis with patchy areas of gadolinium enhancement. Various disease-modifying therapies, including glatiramer acetate, interferon beta1a, and ultimately a course of mitoxantrone were tried, none of which resulted in disease stabilization. Six years ago, she experienced a severe episode of right optic neuritis with minimal recovery despite high-dose IV corticosteroids resulting in marked residual vision impairment limited to light perception only. Several serial MRI studies of the brain have remained unremarkable.

What do you do now?

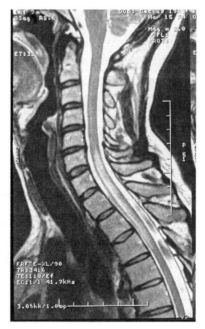

FIGURE 5-1 MRI of the cervical spine demonstrating the characteristic longitudinally extensive intramedullary lesion in a patient with neuromyelitis optica.

In the course of longitudinal clinical follow-up and treatment of patients with MS, it is very important to scrutinize atypical features in individual cases and challenge the diagnosis under these circumstances. Several features of this case are atypical for classical MS, the most striking being a normal MRI of the brain, as well as the longitudinal extent of spinal cord lesions and absence of CSF oligoclonal bands. Additionally, this patient has demonstrated an ongoing poor response to conventional MS disease-modifying therapies. Such features should prompt diagnostic consideration of neuromyelitis optica (NMO).

Until recently, cases of NMO, an idiopathic inflammatory, demyelinating disease of the central nervous system (CNS) that preferentially affects the optic nerves and spinal cord, were commonly misdiagnosed as MS. Such diagnostic confusion has been alleviated by the identification of a diagnostic biomarker for NMO, the serum immunoglobulin G autoantibody, NMO-IgG, which has a specificity and sensitivity of 91% and 73%, respectively, for the disease. Discrimination of NMO from MS is a critical clinical distinction with important therapeutic implications, as these two diseases appear to have different natural histories, prognoses, and therapeutic responses.

Historically, patients with NMO were thought, in general, to have a normal MRI of the brain. Recently, however, brain lesions have been reported in NMO patients, although radiographically these lesions are atypical in appearance and location and do not satisfy diagnostic criteria for classical MS. The NMO antibody's antigenic target is aquaporin 4, a water channel located in the foot processes of astrocytes making up the blood–brain barrier. In approximately 10% of NMO patients, brain lesions are present, but they are unusual for MS and appear to correspond to areas of aquaporin 4 distribution in the CNS, specifically periependymal, periaqueductal, and hypothalamic regions. In addition, large subcortical hemispheric lesions, similar to those seen in posterior reversible leukoencephalopathy syndromes, may occur. Spinal cord lesions in classical MS typically are short (one or two vertebral levels) and often posteriorly located, in contrast to NMO lesions, which are characteristically longitudinally extensive, spanning three or more vertebral segments, and centrally located with gray matter involvement. Other conditions to consider in the differential diagnosis of longitudinally extensive spinal lesions include neurosarcoidosis,

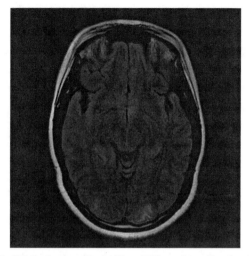

FIGURE 5-2 MRI of the brain of a patient with an NMO spectrum disorder who developed headache, hypertension, and T2/FLAIR hyperintense lesions involving subcortical and juxtacortical white matter hyperintensities, suggestive of posterior reversible leukoencephalopathy.

neoplasms, vascular abnormalities such as dural arterio-venous fistulas, and myelitidies associated with collagen vascular diseases such as systemic lupus erythematosus and Sjögren's syndrome.

CSF in NMO tends to demonstrate a moderate pleocytosis, with neutrophilic rather than lymphocytic preponderance, in addition to elevated protein and abnormal IgG synthesis and index. The presence of CSF oligoclonal bands is much less common in NMO compared to MS.

In 2006, new diagnostic criteria (see below) for NMO were proposed by Wingerchuk and colleagues, which incorporated the NMO-IgG antibody as well as an abnormal MRI of the brain (Fig. 5.2). These criteria require the following:

- Optic neuritis
- Transverse myelitis (typically longitudinally extensive)
- At least two of the following three supportive criteria:
- Brain MRI normal or showing white matter lesions not meeting diagnostic radiologic criteria for MS

- Spinal cord MRI showing lesion extending contiguously over three or more vertebral segments
- NMO-IgG seropositive status

Additionally, NMO can present with unusual brainstem syndromes such as intractable nausea, vomiting and hiccups due to high cervicomedullary lesions. These presentations can be easily confused with gastrointestinal symptomatology, and, therefore, a high index of clinical suspicion for NMO should be maintained in such cases.

Clinically, NMO relapses tend to be more severe, with poor recovery and greater risk of stepwise accrual of disability compared to relapsing-remitting MS exacerbations. Within 5 years of diagnosis, greater than 50% of NMO patients are functionally blind with visual acuity worse than 20/200 or require an assistive device for ambulation. In further contrast to MS, NMO almost uniformly follows a relapsing course, either monophasic or polyphasic, and only rarely has been reported to demonstrate the slow, insidious deterioration characteristic of progressive forms of MS. NMO spectrum disorders, in the form of either relapsing longitudinally extensive transverse myelitidies (LETM) or relapsing optic neuritidies with normal MRI of the brain, have also been described and demonstrate a positive NMO antibody in 50% and up to a third of cases, respectively. Moreover, more than 50% of patients with a first-time episode of LETM and seropositive NMO antibody will have a relapse or convert to definite NMO over the subsequent year, demonstrating that antibody status has predictive implications for disease course.

This patient, with a paucity of brain lesions, a history of bilateral optic neuropathy, and longitudinally extensive cord lesions, has a high likelihood of having NMO, and antibody testing should be performed. Importantly, however, irrespective of antibody status, her clinical presentation formally satisfies diagnostic criteria for NMO.

Regarding future management of this patient, acute exacerbations of NMO are treated similarly to MS attacks with courses of high-dose IV corticosteroids and consideration of rescue plasma exchange for steroid-refractory relapses. IV immunoglobulin is also used anecdotally for acute exacerbations. For attacks involving the brain stem and high cervical lesions, patients should be monitored closely in intensive care units for respiratory compromise. Because of the potential severity of disease, maintenance therapy is critical for the prevention of relapses and disability. Maintenance therapy for NMO generally involves immunosuppressive agents, in contrast to the disease-modifying immunomodulatory agents used in MS. First-line treatments typically include prednisone or steroid-sparing oral immunosuppressants such as azathioprine or mycophenolate mofetil. In patients with severe or frequent attacks, induction therapy with the monoclonal antibody rituximab, which induces B-cell targeted immunosuppression, can be considered. Data regarding the efficacy of the agents are limited, relying on small, uncontrolled, open-label studies. Because of the rarity and severity of the disease, implementation of large-scale, randomized placebo-controlled trials has been unsuccessful. Likewise, there are no data regarding the comparative efficacy of these individual agents in treating NMO for the same reasons. As with MS, patients with NMO are optimally cared for by a multidisciplinary team of MS specialists, nurse practitioners, physiatrists, physical therapists, urologists, psychiatrists, and social workers to best manage their chronic disease course.

KEY POINTS TO REMEMBER

- NMO, an inflammatory, demyelinating disorder of the CNS with a predilection for the optic nerves and spinal cord, is associated with a highly specific serum autoantibody, NMO-IgG, which targets the aquaporin 4 water channel.
- In contrast to MS, NMO tends to spare the brain, manifest longitudinally extensive spinal cord lesions, and cause attacks that are typically more severe than MS exacerbations with greater risk of stepwise disability.
- In contrast to MS, maintenance therapy for NMO involves immunosuppression with prednisone or steroid-sparing immunosuppressants such as azathioprine and mycophenolate mofetil, in addition to the monoclonal antibody rituximab, which induces B-cell specific depletion.

Further Reading

Cree B. Neuromyelitis optica: diagnosis, pathogenesis, and treatment. *Curr Neurol Neurosci Rep* 2008; 8:427-433.

Hazin R, Khan F, Bhatti MT. Neuromyelitis optica: current concepts and prospects for future management. *Curr Opin Ophthalmol* 2009; 20:434-439.

Wingerchuk DM, Weinshenker BG. Neuromyelitis optica. *Curr Treat Options Neurol* 2008; 10:55-66.

6 Pregnancy and Multiple Sclerosis

A 32-year-old woman with relapsing-remitting multiple sclerosis (MS) seeks advice about pregnancy. At age 19 the patient had an episode of optic neuritis with excellent recovery. The diagnosis of MS was made 6 years later when she developed numbness and tingling in her legs, which ascended to the girdle area over 2 weeks. Symptoms resolved completely after a course of intravenous methylprednisolone. Brain MRI showed a modest lesion load, but did meet McDonald criteria for dissemination in space. Treatment was initiated with glatiramer acetate (GA). The patient did well over the next 6 years, during which she got married and completed law school. A recent brain MRI showed one new T2 hyperintense lesion, the first one noted since she began treatment with GA. The patient, whose neurologic examination is normal, indicates that she would like to try to get pregnant in about 9 months, but she has discontinued her oral contraceptive medication.

What do you do now?

Many issues should be considered by a woman—or, preferably by a couple—contemplating having a child. First of all, it is important to emphasize that MS has no known impact on the ability of a woman to conceive. Furthermore, the obstetric outcomes are generally excellent and a recent study (Kelly et al., 2009) demonstrated little difference between the rates of intrauterine growth retardation or cesarean delivery among MS patients compared to the general obstetric population. No increase in other adverse outcomes was observed.

Genetic risk is frequently a concern of patients with MS. MS is considered to be a complex genetic disorder, in which some individuals appear to be at higher risk for developing the disease. The children of a parent with MS are at higher risk for developing MS, but the risk remains low. The lifetime risk for the development of MS in the son of a parent with MS is about 1% and that for a daughter is approximately 4%.

In some situations where a potential parent—man or woman—has significant neurologic impairment and the disease may not be well controlled, other issues should be considered by the couple. Will the patient be physically (and emotionally) capable of providing adequate care for the child? Will the disease affect the economic situation for the parent(s) to the point that it may adversely affect their ability to provide for the child? Fortunately for this patient, these issues do not at this time appear to be a reason for her to avoid having a child.

Women will also be concerned about the potential impact of a pregnancy on their disease. They will be pleased to learn that the risk of relapse is lower during pregnancy than during non-pregnancy periods. However, the potential for an exacerbation is increased during the 3-month postpartum period (Confavreux et al., 1998).

A source of significant concern for a woman with MS is the implication for her disease course if she discontinues her disease-modifying medication while attempting to conceive. Interferon beta preparations carry a Category C pregnancy rating. Although they have not been demonstrated to be teratogenic, interferon has been associated with an increased risk of spontaneous abortion in experimental animals. Hence, its use is contraindicated for women attempting to become pregnant and during pregnancy itself. GA, on the other hand, has been assigned a Category B pregnancy rating, meaning that the agent has not been associated with detrimental effects on the pregnancy or the fetus in humans or in experimental animals. Because of this, it has been this author's practice to discuss with women who are taking GA the potential risks and benefits of remaining on the medication while attempting to conceive and during pregnancy versus those of discontinuing it. The majority of women offered the option of remaining on GA have chosen to do so, but only after receiving the agreement of their obstetrician.

Generally speaking, women who have been off medication during pregnancy should resume treatment as soon as possible after delivery. The results of one study suggested that the administration of intravenous immunoglobulin after delivery decreased the risk of relapse in the postpartum period. However, the existing data are inconclusive and this practice has not been widely adopted.

Another issue for consideration is the question of breastfeeding. Studies have differed on whether breastfeeding has a beneficial effect on the incidence of postpartum relapses, but none have shown a detrimental effect of breastfeeding. Although this author encourages women to breastfeed, he also urges them to discuss with their pediatrician and/or obstetrician the possibility of continuing either interferon or GA while they are lactating. Although no specific data on the safety of interferon beta or GA during breastfeeding are available, these medications are all very large molecules . unlikely to get into breast milk in other than very small quantities.

This case illustrates the fact that physicians should anticipate the possibility that their female patients may desire to become pregnant and should address these issues early. Although this patient did not intend to try to conceive for 9 months, she had discontinued her oral contraceptive and, in fact, became pregnant a few months later. After discussing the issues, she elected to remain on GA and delivered a healthy full-term baby.

KEY POINTS TO REMEMBER

- Many issues should be considered by a woman—or, preferably by a couple—contemplating having a child.
- The obstetric outcomes for women with MS are generally excellent, with little difference from the non-MS population.

- The risk of exacerbations is lower during pregnancy but higher during the postpartum period.
- Interferon therapy should be discontinued before a woman attempts to conceive. Glatiramer acetate has a Category B pregnancy rating, and some physicians discuss with women the option of continuing on the medication while they are attempting to conceive and during the pregnancy.

Further Reading

Achiron A, Kishner I, Dolev M, et al. Effect of intravenous immunoglobulin treatment on pregnancy and postpartum-related relapses in multiple sclerosis. *J Neurol* 2004;251(9):1133–1137.

Confavreux C, Hutchinson M, Hours MM, Cortinovis-Tourniaire P, Moreau T. Rate of pregnancy-related relapse in multiple sclerosis. Pregnancy in Multiple Sclerosis Group. *N Engl J Med.* 1998; 339(5):285–291.

Crabtree-Hartman E. Sex differences in multiple sclerosis. *Continuum: Lifelong Learning Neurol* 2010; 16(5):193–210.

Kelly VM, Nelson LM, Chakraverty EF. Obstetrical outcomes in multiple sclerosis and epilepsy. *Neurology* 2009; 73:1831–1836.

7 Progressive Multifocal Leukoencephalopathy Syndrome and Immune Reconstitution Inflammatory Syndrome

A 32-year-old man with relapsing-remitting multiple sclerosis (MS) was initially treated with subcutaneous interferon beta-1a (IFNB-1a). Five months after starting IFNB he experienced an episode of right optic neuritis, with visual acuity of 20/80 and a central scotoma. Vision recovered well after a course of intravenous methylprednisolone (IVMP), followed by an oral prednisone taper. Four months later, he developed numbness and tingling in his lower extremities and weakness of the right leg that affected his gait. Another course of IVMP was administered and the patient experienced some improvement in his symptoms but was left with mild residual weakness of his leg. Brain MRI showed extensive T2 hyperintense lesions, with four new gadolinium-enhancing lesions. Cervical spine MRI showed a gadolinium-enhancing lesion at C4. Treatment with IFNB was discontinued and natalizumab therapy was initiated, with intravenous infusions administered every 4 weeks.

The patient tolerated the natalizumab infusions well and experienced no relapses over the next 12 months.

A repeat brain MRI showed no new lesions and resolution of the previously seen gadolinium enhancement. The patient was employed as a high school history teacher and had no limitations in his activities of daily living, except for mild gait abnormality that limited his ability to walk long distances. At a visit 18 months after the initiation of natalizumab therapy the patient's wife reported that her husband had seemed to be particularly irritable over the previous few weeks and that she had noticed he seemed to have some difficulty finding words. The patient himself reported no new concerns. On neurologic examination, the mental status was normal except for the presence of mild anomia. Mild weakness of the right upper extremity was detected, in addition to the previously noted paresis of the right leg.

What do you do now?

This patient has classical relapsing-remitting MS. He was appropriately initiated on IFNB-1a as disease-modifying therapy. Unfortunately, he had recurrent breakthrough disease with relapses involving optic neuritis and partial myelitis. Because of this suboptimal response, the treatment was changed to natalizumab. After 18 months of treatment, the patient developed relatively subtle symptoms of personality change and word-finding difficulty, as well as new weakness of the right arm. These events occurring in a patient on natalizumab should definitely raise concern about the possibility of progressive multifocal leukoencephalopathy (PML), and investigations should be initiated immediately.

Could the patient be experiencing new MS activity? This is certainly possible but seems relatively unlikely. Personality change due to MS is uncommon, although it may be misinterpreted as such in the context of depression, which does occur frequently in the disease. Irritability is sometimes encountered in patients taking interferon, but it is not a feature of natalizumab therapy. Language disturbance, including true word-finding difficulty or anomia, is distinctly uncommon in MS. Of course, it is important to distinguish aphasia from dysarthria, which is common in MS. A hemiparetic pattern of weakness certainly occurs in MS but is much less common than paraparesis. In addition, the temporal profile of the new symptomatology is not characteristic for MS relapses, in which new symptoms generally come on over a matter of days.

In contrast, this case scenario is strongly suggestive of PML, an opportunistic viral infection of the CNS caused by the polyoma virus known as JC virus. PML for many years has been principally associated with HIV infection (occurring in up to 5% of such patients) and, to a much lesser extent, in people with hematologic malignancies. PML is now a well-recognized, albeit infrequent, consequence of prolonged exposure to natalizumab in MS patients. It tends to present in a subacute manner. Although symptoms and signs of PML can mimic those of MS, personality change, cognitive dysfunction, and language disturbance, as well as hemiparesis, are common early findings in PML. In contrast, involvement of the optic nerves or spinal cord, frequent sites of involvement in MS, rarely, if ever, occurs.

PML is significantly related to the duration of exposure to natalizumab. Only one case has so far been reported with fewer than 12 infusions. With over 83,000 patients exposed to the drug worldwide, as of July 5, 2011, 145 patients with PML had been identified after a mean exposure of 17.9 months. The overall risk for PML was 1.62 per 1,000 patients (CI 1.37–1.91). However, the incidence for all patients receiving drug for at least 12 months was 2.41 (2.04-2.84), increasing to 3.03 (2.51-3.62) for all those on the medication for 24 months or more. The peak incidence was for patients in the treatment epoch between 25 and 36 infusions, for whom the incidence rate was 1.96 (1.52–2.43). Thus far, the incidence rate does not appear to be increasing beyond that duration of exposure.

As soon as the suspicion of PML arises, further therapy with natalizumab should be halted. MRI of the brain should be obtained (Figs. 7-1 and 7-2). The appearance of any new brain lesions on MRI obtained after 6 months of natalizumab treatment should raise the question of PML. Although similarity to the appearance of MS lesions on MRI may occur, several specific features of MRI in PML occur, as reported by Boster et al. (2009). Large confluent T2 hyperintense lesions occur commonly in PML but rarely in MS (74% vs. 2%, $p < 0.0001$). Deep gray matter lesions were also more frequent in PML (31% vs. 7%, $p < 0.001$). In addition, crescentic cerebellar lesions were seen only in PML Although classically PML has been associated with the absence of gadolinium enhancement, this is not the case in

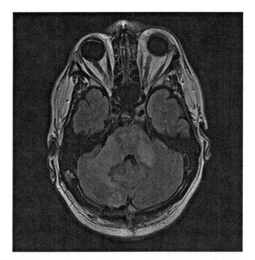

FIGURE 7-1 MRI FLAIR sequence showing large coalescent lesions in both cerebellar hemispheres that were proven on biopsy to be PML. The patient had been on natalizumab for approximately 2 years.

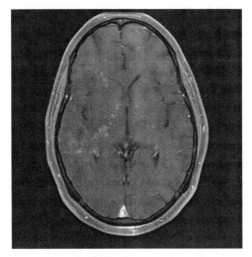

FIGURE 7-2 Gadolinium-enhanced T1 images from the same patient depicted in Figure 7.1 showing innumerable small enhancing lesions believed to be due to the immune response inflammatory syndrome (IRIS).

natalizumab-associated PML: in one report, gadolinium enhancement was observed in 43% of 28 cases of PML at the time of diagnosis.

CSF should be examined and sent for polymerase chain reaction (PCR) testing for JC virus DNA. It is important to note that many commercial laboratories doing JC PCR are not capable of detecting the low number of copies that are often present in natalizumab-associated PML. Clifford et al. (2010) reported that 16 of 28 cases had fewer than 500 copies, and sometimes very low copy numbers are present.

When PML is diagnosed or strongly suspected, current recommendations advise that patients be treated with plasma exchange (PLEX) or immunoabsorption to speed the clearance of the monoclonal antibody and restore immunologic function. No specific drug therapy has been demonstrated to be effective in ameliorating the disease.

After natalizumab is withdrawn, and perhaps accentuated by PLEX or immunoabsorption therapy, an immune reconstitution inflammatory syndrome (IRIS) invariably develops, typically becoming recognizable a few weeks after cessation of the monoclonal antibody. This happens also in the context of HIV, but it is typically less severe in that setting. IRIS in natalizumab-associated PML is typically characterized by neurologic worsening, which is usually transient but may be severe or even fatal. It is accompanied by increased brain swelling, which may be associated with increased intracranial pressure and headache. During IRIS, the brain MRI often shows enlargement of the lesion(s) with prominent edema and usually with gadolinium enhancement. Treatment with high-dose IVMP should be given in the setting of IRIS and appears to be beneficial in reducing brain swelling and neurologic deterioration. Some have suggested that steroids be administered prophylactically at the time of PML diagnosis to lessen the development of IRIS. Of the PML cases reported by Clifford et al. (2010), only 8 of 28 were fatal, resulting in a survival rate of 71%, albeit in many instances with severe neurologic disability.

Continuing work is attempting to identify ways to lessen the risks of PML in the natalizumab-treated MS population. Recent work, using a particular assay for JC virus antibody, suggests that the risk for PML may be extremely low for individuals who are antibody negative. If these data are confirmed, the use of natalizumab for the treatment of MS could be significantly modified. In the meantime, a search for effective therapy for PML continues.

KEY POINTS TO REMEMBER

- PML is now a well-recognized, albeit infrequent, consequence of prolonged exposure to natalizumab in MS patients.
- Although symptoms and signs of PML can mimic those of MS, personality change, cognitive dysfunction, and language disturbance, as well as hemiparesis, are common early findings in PML.
- As soon as the suspicion of PML arises, further therapy with natalizumab should be halted. MRI of the brain should be obtained. The appearance of any new brain lesions on MRI obtained after 6 months of natalizumab treatment should raise the question of PML.
- When PML is diagnosed or strongly suspected, current recommendations advise that patients be treated with plasma exchange (PLEX) or immunoabsorption to speed the clearance of the monoclonal antibody and restore immunologic function.

- After natalizumab is withdrawn, and perhaps accentuated by PLEX or immunoabsorption therapy, an immune reconstitution inflammatory syndrome (IRIS) invariably develops, typically becoming recognizable a few weeks after cessation of the monoclonal antibody.

Further Reading

Boster A, Hreha S, Berger JR, et al. Progressive multifocal leukoencephalopathy and relapsing-remitting multiple sclerosis: a comparative study. *Arch Neurol* 2009; 66(5):593-599.

Clifford DB, De Luca A, Simpson DM, Arendt G, Giovannoni G, Nath A. Natalizumab-associated progressive multifocal leukoencephalopathy in patients with multiple sclerosis: lessons from 28 cases. *Lancet Neurol* 2010; 9(4):438-446.

Gorelik L, Lerner M, Bixler S, et al. Anti-JC virus antibodies: implications for PML risk stratification. *Ann Neurol* 2010; 68(3):295-303.

Warnke C, Menge T, Hartung HP, et al. Natalizumab and progressive multifocal leukoencephalopathy: what are the causal factors and can it be avoided? *Arch Neurol* 2010; 67(8):923-930.

8   Neuroborreliosis

A 47-year-old otherwise healthy man presents with a two-day history of headaches, low-grade fever, and chills. He is the owner of a summer camp in southern Connecticut. In addition, he has been experiencing "heaviness" involving the left side of his face, which he likens to a "Novocaine" injection for a dental procedure. Several counselors and campers have remarked that the left side of his face appears droopy. He denies any associated upper respiratory symptoms or contact with any other ill persons. He denies any insect bites or rashes at present but had a tick bite about 2 months ago with associated bull's-eye rash, for which he was diagnosed with Lyme disease and treated with a course of oral doxycycline. On examination, he has a temperature of 101.3 but no nuchal rigidity. Neurologic examination is significant for a left peripheral seventh-nerve palsy and bilaterally brisk reflexes with silent plantar responses. An MRI of the brain demonstrates a few small nonspecific subcortical T2 hyperintense lesions without gadolinium enhancement. CSF analysis reveals a moderate lymphocytic pleocytosis with slightly elevated protein and the presence of oligoclonal bands that are absent in the serum. Viral PCRs and cultures were negative. CSF *B. burgdorferi* IgM antibody is elevated.

What do you do now?

The neurologic complications of Lyme disease are multiple, varied, and easily confused with other infectious and inflammatory conditions, making diagnosis difficult and sometimes controversial, particularly if there is no clear evidence of previous exposure or infection by the tick-borne spirochete *Borrelia burgdorferi*. Clinical suspicion is certainly heightened in this case by the history of a typical bull's-eye–shaped erythema chronicum migrans rash, which is present in 60% to 80% of patients. Other organ systems that can be affected include the musculoskeletal system, with monoarthritides and polyarthrides, and the nervous system, which is involved in approximately 10% to 15% of infected persons in both the United States and Europe. Additionally, cardiac manifestations such as dysrhythmias and conduction block can occur.

To support a diagnosis of neuroborreliosis, there should be evidence of possible exposure to bites by *Ixodes* ticks, clinical findings suggestive of neurologic manifestations of Lyme disease, and positive laboratory studies, including serologies with or without the presence of CSF Lyme antibodies. Clinically, Lyme disease is characterized as presenting in three stages: early or acute localized disease, early disseminated, and late disseminated disease. Nervous system involvement generally reflects disseminated disease and early in the course can include cranial neuropathies, typically unilateral or bilateral peripheral seventh-nerve (Bell's) palsies, in addition to lymphocytic meningitis, radiculoneuritis, and, less commonly, optic neuritis and acute inflammatory demyelinating polyneuropathy or Guillain-Barré syndrome. Later manifestations include encephalomyelitis and peripheral neuropathy. Lyme encephalomyelitis is often considered in the differential diagnosis for multiple sclerosis (MS) and can create a diagnostic dilemma not easily resolved. In such a clinical scenario, patients may receive a course of intravenous antibiotics for neuroborreliosis, but thereafter, if any additional clinical or radiographic activity occurs, they may ultimately be diagnosed and treated for MS.

Acute neurologic involvement usually occurs weeks to several months after a tick bite. Consistent with this temporal relationship, this patient presents two months after initial skin inoculation with left-sided peripheral seventh-nerve (facial) palsy in the setting of a lymphocytic meningitis. Lymphocytic meningitis accompanied by cranial nerve or radicular involvement is considered the most common form of CNS Lyme disease. A small percentage of Lyme lymphocytic meningitis cases occur in isolation without associated cranial neuropathy. Presenting symptoms tend to resemble a viral, aseptic meningitis with fever, headache, neck stiffness, and photophobia, although the presentation tends to be less acute than viral meningitides. Seventh-nerve (facial) palsy is the most commonly reported cranial neuropathy associated with Lyme, occurring in approximately 8% of cases, as confirmed by the Centers for Disease Control and Prevention. Other cranial nerves less commonly affected include oculomotor, trochlear and abducens, vestibulocochlear, and trigeminal. Retrospective studies suggest that optic neuritis is exceedingly rare. The most common form of neuroborreliosis in Europe is a lymphocytic meningoradiculitis, otherwise known as Garin-Bujadoux-Bannwarth's syndrome, which is rare in the United States.

Serological testing for Lyme involves a two-tier approach with initial screening enzyme-linked immunoabsorbent assay (ELISA) followed by confirmatory Western blot. During the initial 4 to 6 weeks after exposure patients can be seronegative due to inadequate mounting of an initial immune response. CSF analysis typically demonstrates a moderate pleocytosis between 100 and 200 cells with moderately elevated protein and normal glucose. A negative test for Lyme antibodies in the CSF does not exclude neuroborreliosis, and the presence of *B. burgdorferi* antibodies in the CSF does not itself establish a diagnosis, as antibodies can, to a limited extent, diffuse from the serum to CSF. Proof requires detection of a greater level of antibodies in the CSF compared to the serum. CSF Lyme PCR is an alternative method of testing but carries a low sensitivity because of the presence of small numbers of organisms in spinal fluid. CSF analysis should include diagnostic testing for other possible causes of aseptic meningitis, such as West Nile, herpes simplex, and enteroviruses.

Standard treatment of neuroborreliosis involves parenteral antibiotics, specifically ceftriaxone or penicillin, for 2 to 4 weeks. In penicillin- or cephalosporin-allergic patients, alternatives include tetracycline or chloramphenicol. The use of concomitant courses of high-dose corticosteroids depends on the clinical setting and extent of CNS inflammation. Serial CSF analysis should be performed after the 2- to 4-week treatment period to assess the need for continuation of therapy, and thereafter at 6 months. Persistent pleocytosis suggests the need for retreatment with antibiotics, in contrast to elevation of CSF antibodies, which can persist for long periods and not necessarily reflect ongoing active infection.

KEY POINTS TO REMEMBER

- Neurologic involvement of Lyme disease occurs only in disseminated disease.
- Acute presentation of lymphocytic meningitis, cranial neuropathy (primarily facial palsy), and radiculoneuritis represents the classic triad of acute, early neuroborreliosis, typically presenting weeks to months after the inciting *Ixodes* tick bite.
- A diagnosis of neuroborreliosis should be made with caution in seronegative patients, with the exception of the first 4 to 6 weeks after the inciting *Ixodes* tick bite, when serum antibodies may be absent.
- CSF and serum evaluation for synthesis of anti-*Borrelia burgdorferi* antibodies can be informative in the proper clinical context, but PCR for *B. burgdorferi* is of extremely limited utility.

Further Reading

Halperin JJ. Nervous system Lyme disease. *Infect Dis Clin North Am* 2008; 22:261.

Marques A. Chronic Lyme disease: a review. *Infect Dis Clin North Am* 2008; 22:341.

Rupprecht TA, Koedel U, Fingerle V, et al. The pathogenesis of Lyme neuroborreliosis: from infection to inflammation. *Mol Med* 2008; 14:205.

HTLV Myelopathy

A 48-year-old taxi driver presents with a two-year history of progressive lower extremity weakness and achy lower back pain. In addition, he reports associated lower extremity stiffness, burning paresthesias, and urinary dysfunction for the past several months. Past medical history is significant for lumbar degenerative disc disease diagnosed one year ago, for which he underwent an L4-5 laminectomy without any significant postoperative improvement. He takes no medications. He smokes one pack of cigarettes daily and drinks about two beers on the weekends. He works as a taxi driver and previously worked for the American Red Cross transporting blood products in the 1970s. He was born and lives in New York City and rarely travels outside the country. There is no family history of known neurologic or autoimmune diseases, including multiple sclerosis (MS).

On examination, he is a well-appearing man of normal habitus. General examination is significant for several tattoos on his forearms. Mental status is intact. Speech is clear and fluent without language deficits, and cranial nerve examination is intact apart from some subtle pallor to his left optic disc. Motor examination demonstrates normal tone and full power in the upper extremities. Lower extremities demonstrate moderate spasticity with mild weakness of 4+/5 with hip and knee flexion. Deep tendon reflexes are brisk 3+ symmetric with bilaterally extensor plantar responses. Sensory examination demonstrates diminished vibration in the toes bilaterally and patchy loss of pinprick over the mid-torso without a defined sensory level. Coordination testing reveals difficulty with heel-knee-shin testing secondary to lower extremity weakness without clear dystaxia. Gait is slow and mildly spastic and paraparetic. An MRI spine survey demonstrates multiple patchy intramedullary white matter abnormalities throughout the cervicothoracic spinal cord without gadolinium enhancement. Laboratory studies including ESR, B12, folate, methylmalonic acid, TSH, Lyme, and ANA are normal. HIV testing is negative. An MRI of the brain demonstrates a few nonspecific white matter lesions without periventricular or callosal involvement. CSF analysis demonstrates 3 white blood cells, elevated protein of 70, negative cultures, negative CSF VDRL, positive oligoclonal bands, and normal IgG synthesis. CSF cytology is normal. HTLV-1 serology comes back positive.

What do you do now?

The patient presents with symptoms of slowly worsening bilateral lower extremity weakness and dysesthesias accompanied by urinary dysfunction with an examination revealing spastic paraparesis, distal vibratory loss, and a suspended sensory level to pinprick in the thoracic region. Clinically, the patient's presentation is highly suspicious for spinal cord pathology, specifically a chronic, progressive myelopathy. The differential diagnosis for a progressive myelopathy is lengthy and several etiologies should be considered, including demyelinating, infectious, degenerative, inflammatory, toxic-metabolic, vascular, and neoplastic. A detailed review of systems often provides helpful clues to the etiology of the myelopathy and can assist in tailoring the battery of laboratory investigations. For example, are there systemic stigmata of infection, collagen vascular disease, risk factors for vitamin deficiency, recent trauma, constitutional symptoms to suggest a neoplastic etiology, or a family history of neurologic disease? Important conditions to consider include primary progressive MS, subacute combined degeneration, spinal cord tumors or vascular abnormalities, primary lateral sclerosis, hereditary spastic paraplegias, HIV vacuolar myelopathy, and other infectious as well as collagen vascular diseases, such as Sjogren's syndrome.

An MRI of the cervicothoracic spine with and without contrast should be performed to evaluate for intrinsic cord pathology or extrinsic, compressive processes affecting the cord. Intrinsic white matter lesions involving the cord are suspicious for demyelinating disease and warrant a follow-up MRI of the brain. Radiographic findings suspicious for demyelination in conjunction with a history of progressive myelopathy raise suspicion for primary progressive MS. An important consideration in making a diagnosis of any form of MS is the absence of any better explanation for presenting symptomatology and paraclinical findings. The differential diagnosis for primary progressive MS is also lengthy and includes mimickers for a progressive spastic paraparesis such as cervical or lumbar degenerative disc disease, subacute combined degeneration secondary to B12 or copper deficiency states, hereditary spastic paraparesis, copper deficiency myelopathy, vascular cord lesions such as arteriovenous fistulas, lymphoma, and tropical spastic paraparesis/HTLV-1/2–associated myelopathy (TSP/HAM). While our patient does not live in a region where HTLV is endemic (Japan, Africa, Caribbean, and South America), he does carry a risk factor for HTLV, specifically his handling of blood products in the 1970s, prior to the institution of standardized screening procedures for blood-borne viruses in 1988.

Over 90% of individuals with incidental HTLV-1 seropositivity are asymptomatic carriers, with a lifetime risk of developing HAM/TSP of less than 1%. The majority of patients, approximately 60%, present clinically with a slow, insidious progression of lower extremity weakness and spasticity, in addition to low back pain and urinary and erectile dysfunction. Relapsing, remitting features are considered uncharacteristic. The average age of onset is in the third to fourth decade. Anatomically, HTLV myelopathy has a predilection for the anterolateral corticospinal tracts of the thoracic spinal cord. The pathogenesis of the disease remains unclear, but lesions demonstrate a T-cell–mediated inflammatory process with fibrosis and neurodegeneration. The neurologic sequelae of latent HTLV infection can occur decades after initial serocoversion, although typically symptoms present within 3 years of infection. HTLV-1 infection has also been associated with T-cell leukemia.

Effective therapeutic options for HTLV myelopathy are limited and based on small open-label studies of various immunotherapies. Generally, treatment focuses on symptomatic management of pain, spasticity, and urinary dysfunction. Therapies that have been used in an effort to slow progression of the disease include corticosteroids, plasmapheresis, danazol, and immunosuppressants such as cyclophosphamide and alpha interferon. Prognosis for HTLV myelopathy is overall poor. with a majority of patients requiring assistive devices for ambulation within 10 years of diagnosis and becoming wheelchair-bound after two decades. It is therefore critical to counsel patients seropositive for HTLV-1 infection to use barrier-method contraception and abstain from breastfeeding and blood donation to avoid transmitting the virus to uninfected individuals.

KEY POINTS TO REMEMBER

- HTLV-1-associated myelopathy/tropical spastic paraparesis (HAM/TSP) typically involves the thoracolumbar spinal cord and is clinically characterized by symmetric spasticity, lower extremity weakness, bladder dysfunction, and pain.

- Over 90% of individuals with incidental HTLV-1 seropositivity are asymptomatic carriers, with a lifetime risk of developing HAM/TSP of less than 1%.
- The differential diagnosis of HAM/TSP includes progressive MS, primary lateral sclerosis, hereditary spastic paraplegias, subacute combined degeneration, HIV vacuolar myelopathy, and other infectious as well as collagen vascular diseases, such as Sjôgren's syndrome, with associated myelopathies.
- No therapy has been conclusively demonstrated to prevent the long-term disability associated with HAM/TSP; however, clinical improvements have been reported in open-label studies of corticosteroids, plasmapheresis, danazol, immunosuppressants, and alpha interferon.

Further Reading

Cooper SA, van der Loeff MS, Taylor GP. The neurology of HTLV-1 infection. *Pract Neurol* 2009; 9:16-26.

Matsuura E, Yamano Y, Jacobson S. Neuroimmunity of HTLV-1 infection. *J Neuroimmune Pharmacol* 2010; 5:310-325.

Oh U, Jacobson S. Treatment of HTLV-1-associated myelopathy/tropical spastic paraparesis: towards rational targeted therapy. *Neurol Clin* 2008; 26(3):781.

10 Varicella Zoster Myelopathy

A 46-year-old otherwise healthy woman with a recent history of a painful vesicular rash involving her right lateral chest 6 weeks ago presents to her primary care physician (PCP) with symptoms of left leg weakness and burning paresthesias in addition to urinary retention. She had received a two-week course of oral valacyclovir for the herpes zoster rash, with gradual healing of vesicles and moderate post-herpetic neuralgia. Her PCP refers her for neurologic evaluation, and on examination she is found to have a sensory level to pinprick at the T6 dermatome, mild weakness involving her left hip and knee flexors, preponderantly brisk left patellar and ankle jerk reflexes, with an extensor left plantar response. An MRI of the thoracic spine is obtained, which demonstrates a gadolinium-enhancing T2 hyperintense lesion at the left T4 level. CSF studies demonstrate a moderate mononuclear pleocytosis with normal protein. Polymerase chain reaction (PCR) for varicella zoster virus (VZV) DNA is negative; however, titers for anti-VZV IgM and IgG are elevated. She is diagnosed with suspected zoster myelitis and admitted to the inpatient hospital service for further management.

What do you do now?

VZV is a human neurotropic herpesvirus whose primary infection causes varicella or chickenpox, with subsequent potential latency along the entire neuraxis, including cranial nerve, dorsal root, and autonomic ganglia. Immunocompromised states, such as age extremes, HIV/AIDS, cancer, and treatment with immunosuppressants, strongly predispose to VZV reactivation with a wide variety of potential neurologic manifestations, including herpes zoster, meningoencephalitis, polyradiculoneuritis, vasculopathy, retinopathy, cerebellitis, and myelopathy. The pathologic process responsible for neurologic sequelae of VZV is uncertain, but either direct invasion or vasculitic involvement has been implicated.

Roughly 25% to 40% of cases of transverse myelitis are attributed to viral infections. The frequency of transverse myelitis accompanying or subsequent to VZV infection is approximately 0.3%. Two clinical presentations have been described. Firstly, in immunocompetent patients, VZV myelitis presents as a self-limiting monophasic spastic paraparesis accompanied by initial sensory dysfunction and impaired sphincteric function. Typically, this is a post-infectious entity, occurring on average approximately two weeks after an acute case of zoster infection, although importantly VZV myelitis may occur in the absence of rash, a condition known as zoster sine herpete. The diagnosis of any neurologic complication of VZV in the absence of rash requires the presence of VZV DNA or anti-VZV antibody, or both, in the CSF. Clinically, neurologic deficits present with ipsilateral involvement of the spinal segments of the affected dermatome. In the majority of patients with VZV myelitis, neurologic deficits are unilateral; when bilateral, they are typically asymmetric, with corticospinal and posterior column deficits presenting ipsilateral and spinothalamic findings contralateral to the rash, respectively. CSF studies generally disclose a mild mononuclear pleocytosis with elevated or normal protein. This presentation is generally self-limited, and patients may demonstrate improvement either spontaneously or after a course of intravenous antiviral therapy with high-dose corticosteroids.

In immunocompromised patients, VZV myelitis presents in a much more insidious, aggressive, and potentially fatal manner. Imaging studies typically demonstrate multiple lesions not restricted to a single vertebral level, with variable amounts of edema and enhancement. Longitudinally extensive lesions have been described; therefore, VZV myelopathy should be considered in the differential diagnosis of entities such as intramedullary neurosarcoidosis, spinal cord tumors, and seronegative neuromyelitis optica syndromes. Cases of spinal cord infarction secondary to VZV vasculopathy have also been described with demonstration of abnormalities involving diffusion-weighted imaging.

There is no standard-of-care treatment regimen for VZV myelitis. It is a challenging diagnosis, and early therapeutic intervention with antiviral therapy using intravenous acyclovir appears to have a significant effect on optimizing outcomes and preventing residual neurologic sequelae. Maintaining a high index of clinical suspicion, therefore, is critical. Concomitant use of intravenous high-dose corticosteroids is of unclear benefit but may help reduce the duration of acute neuritis. Adjunct corticosteroids, however, are often used in combination with antiviral coverage to avoid fostering dissemination of viral infection and recrudescence.

KEY POINTS TO REMEMBER

- VZV myelitis is rare in immunocompetent patients and can present in the absence of the typical zoster vesicular rash (zoster sine herpete).
- Detection of VZV DNA and anti-VZV antibodies in the CSF is considered pathognomonic for VZV myelitis.
- A high index of clinical suspicion is critical to making the diagnosis of VZV myelitis and initiating appropriate antiviral therapy early on to optimize prognosis.

Further Reading
Devinsky O, Cho ES, Petito CK, et al. Herpes zoster myelitis. *Brain* 1991; 114:1181-1196.
Gilden DH, Beinlich BR, Rubinstein EM, et al. Varicella-zoster myelitis: an expanding spectrum. *Neurology* 1994; 44:1818-1823.
Mueller NH, Gilden DH, Cohrs RJ, et al. Varicella zoster virus infection: clinical features, molecular pathogenesis of disease, and latency. *Neurol Clin* 2008; 28(3):675.

11 Antiphospholipid Antibody Syndrome

A 30-year-old woman developed "numbness" of her left arm that spread over several days to involve the left side of her neck, torso, and leg. Her gait was not affected and she did not have functional impairment of her left arm She initially consulted her primary care physician, who ordered some blood tests. These came back normal, except for a weakly positive antinuclear antibody test. Because of this result, he referred the patient to a rheumatologist, as well as to a neurologist.

The patient has no prior neurologic history or any significant medical illnesses. She takes no medication except an oral contraceptive. She is married and has never been pregnant, but she and her husband now wish to begin a family.

On neurologic examination, the patient had no objective signs, though she was complaining of "tingling" on the left side. The general medical examination was normal. Brain MRI demonstrated a 1-cm enhancing lesion in the right dorsal pons and two tiny T2 hyperintense lesions in the cerebral white matter. Cervical spinal cord MRI was normal.

The rheumatologist ordered additional blood tests, which were normal with the exception of an elevated anticardiolipin antibody IgG at a titer of 1:23 and an antiphosphatidyl serine antibody titer of 1:100. The rheumatologist tells the patient she has anticardiolipin antibody syndrome (ACAS) and recommends that she begin treatment with aspirin 325 mg daily.

What do you do now?

From a neurologist's point of view, the vexing question sometimes arises as to whether a patient has multiple sclerosis (MS) or manifestations of ACAS. In this patient, the physician should approach the case by asking whether the patient satisfies criteria for ACAS. The current diagnosis is based on the updated Sapporo criteria, which require clinical evidence of either vascular thrombosis or pregnancy morbidity (Table 11-1). The former is characterized by one or more clinical episodes, in any organ, of arterial, venous, or small vessel thrombosis. To satisfy the criterion of pregnancy morbidity, a woman should experience (a) one or more unexplained deaths of a morphologically normal fetus at >10 weeks' gestation; (b) one or more premature births of a morphologically normal baby before the 34th week of gestation because of eclampsia, severe preeclampsia, or placental insufficiency; or (c) three or more unexplained consecutive spontaneous abortions before the 10th week of gestation. One or more of the following laboratory criteria must be satisfied:

1. Lupus anticoagulant present in plasma on at least two occasions a minimum of 12 weeks apart
2. Anticardiolipin antibody (IgG and/or IgM) in plasma or serum in medium or high titer (>1:40) or >99th percentile on at least two occasions a minimum of 12 weeks apart
3. Anti-β_2 glycoprotein I antibody (IgG and/or IgM) in titer >99th percentile on at least two occasions a minimum of 12 weeks apart.

Definite diagnosis of ACAS requires the presence of at least one clinical criterion and at least one laboratory criterion. One should avoid making a definitive diagnosis if the time between the clinical manifestation and the demonstration antiphospholipid antibody titer is less than 12 weeks or more than 5 years.

A difficulty confronting the clinician is the need to determine whether lesions on a cranial MRI represent an ischemic process or some other pathology such as inflammation/demyelination. In making that judgment one must consider the location and distribution of lesions, the shape of the lesions, and the presence and nature of enhancement after contrast administration. Acute ischemic lesions should demonstrate abnormalities on diffusion-weighted imaging.

Clinical Criteria
- Vascular thrombosis
  I. One or more clinical episodes of arterial, venous, or small vessel thrombosis in any tissue or organ. Thrombosis must be confirmed via imaging, Doppler studies, or histopathology, with the exception of superficial venous thrombosis.
- Pregnancy morbidity
  I. One or more unexplained deaths of a morphologically normal fetus at or beyond the 10th week of gestation with normal fetal morphology documented by ultrasound or examination

  Or

  II. One or more premature births of a morphologically normal neonate at or before the 34th week of gestation because of preeclampsia or severe placental insufficiency

  Or

  III. Three or more unexplained consecutive spontaneous abortions before the 10th week of gestation with maternal anatomic or hormonal abnormalities and exclusion of maternal and paternal chromosomal causes
- Laboratory criteria
  I. Anticardiolipin antibody of immunoglobulin (Ig) G and/or IgM isotype and measured by a standardized enzyme-linked immunoabsorbent assay or anti-b2-glycoprotein 1 of IgG and/or IgM isotype in blood, present in medium or high titer, on two or more occasions 12 weeks or more apart
  II. Lupus anticoagulant present in plasma on two or more occasions 12 weeks or more apart and detected according to the guidelines of the International Society of Thrombosis and Hemostasis, in the following steps:
     A. Demonstration of a prolonged phospholipid-dependent coagulation screening test (eg, activated partial thromboplastin time, Kaolin clotting time, dilute Russell's viper venom time, dilute prothrombin time, Textarin time)
     B. Failure to correct the prolonged screening test by mixing with normal platelet-poor plasma
     C. Shortening or correction of the prolonged screening test by the addition of excess phospholipid
     D. Exclusion of other coagulopathies as appropriate (eg, factor VIII inhibitor, heparin)

Data from Miyakis S, Lockshin MD, Atsumi T, et al. International consensus statement on an update of the classification criteria for definite antiphospholipid syndrome. *J Thromb Haemost* 2006; 4(2):295-306.

Demyelinating lesions typically have characteristic patterns meeting criteria for "dissemination in space," as described in detail in Chapter 1. In cases that do not look distinctively like MS, additional data must be sought. Imaging the spinal cord, particularly the cervical region, can be very helpful. Vascular disease seldom involves the cervical spinal cord, whereas MS commonly does. Examination of the CSF may also be helpful. Although oligoclonal bands and elevated IgG index occasionally occur in ACAS, these findings are much more likely in patients with MS.

The MRI of this patient does not satisfy criteria for dissemination in space. Nonetheless, the location of the pontine lesion is very atypical for a vascular lesion and the pattern of gadolinium enhancement was not typical. Because of the uncertainty, lumbar puncture is warranted.

In this patient, the diagnosis of ACAS was not justified because only one set of serologic observations has been obtained and the titer of antiphospholipid antibody was not high enough to warrant the diagnosis. In addition, the neurologic episode was unlikely to be of vascular origin in view of its tempo, characterized by gradual onset of symptoms, as well as its imaging features.

Neurologic manifestations of ACAS are predominantly ischemic. These may be primarily arterial thromboses, but cardioembolic events may also occur as ACAS not infrequently affects the heart, particularly with valvular involvement. In addition, venous thromboses may involve the cerebral veins or venous sinuses. The former may result in venous infarction and the latter may, at times, result in raised intracranial pressure. Of course, the occurrence of venous thrombosis in the leg veins may be associated with paradoxical cerebral embolization through a patent foramen ovale or other abnormality leading to right-to-left shunting.

The management of cerebral thrombotic events in the setting of ACAS generally mirrors that in patients without ACAS. Close attention to the management of other vascular risk factors such as hypertension, hyperlipidemia, and smoking is important. Prophylactic treatment with antiplatelet agents is indicated.

Thrombocytopenia is another frequent manifestation of ACAS. When severe this can be associated with intracerebral or subarachnoid hemorrhage. In addition, the recommended management of venous thrombosis in the setting of ACAS is moderate-intensity anticoagulation. This treatment, of course, also subjects the patient to the increased risk of intracranial bleeding.

Based on a randomized clinical trial, the prophylactic treatment of asymptomatic patients with anticardiolipin antibodies or lupus anticoagulant with antiplatelet agents does not appear warranted. Of course, it is always prudent to vigorously address additional cardiovascular risk factors.

Rarely, a catastrophic ACAS (also known as Hughes syndrome) occurs, marked by the development of microthrombi in multiple organs. This can result in multiple organ failure. The condition is sometimes triggered by infection, trauma, surgery, or withdrawal of anticoagulation. Although no randomized trials have been conducted for this very uncommon condition, intensive anticoagulation is generally recommended (in the absence of hemorrhage), often in conjunction with the administration of high-dose glucocorticoids. Plasmapheresis or intravenous immunoglobulin has been suggested for use in refractory cases.

KEY POINTS TO REMEMBER

- The diagnosis of ACAS requires clinical criteria of either vascular thrombosis or pregnancy morbidity.
- The diagnosis of ACAS also requires laboratory abnormalities, consisting of either lupus anticoagulant, substantial elevation of anticardiolipin antibody, or elevation of β2 microglobulin antibody. Whatever abnormality is used as the criterion must be present on at least two occasions a minimum of 12 weeks apart.
- The management of vascular events in ACAS is similar to that in patients without the syndrome. The prophylactic use of antiplatelet antibodies in asymptomatic patients with anticardiolipin antibodies does not appear warranted.
- Rarely, a catastrophic ACAS (Hughes syndrome) occurs, characterized by the development of microthrombi in multiple organs.

Further Reading

Cervera R. Update on the diagnosis, treatment, and prognosis of the catastrophic antiphospholipid syndrome. *Curr Rheumatol Rep* 2010; 12(1):70-76.

Giannakopoulos B, Krilis SA. How I treat the antiphospholipid syndrome. *Blood* 2009; 114(10):2020-2030.

Mayer M, Cerovec M, Rados M, Cikes N. Antiphospholipid syndrome and central nervous system. *Clin Neurol Neurosurg* 2010; 112(7):602-608.

Ruiz-Irastorza G, Crowther M, Branch W, Khamashta MA. Antiphospholipid syndrome. *Lancet* 2010; 376(9751):1498-1509.

12 Rheumatoid Arthritis

A 45-year-old woman has a 15-year history of rheumatoid arthritis (RA). Because of continued joint pain and swelling, despite the use of nonsteroidal anti-inflammatory drugs and low-dose methotrexate, she was switched to etanercept, which she has been taking for a year. On that regimen, she has experienced significant improvement in her joint symptoms. She has been experiencing headache and neck pain for approximately 9 months. During that time, she has also noted pain in her left thumb and index and middle fingers, as well as numbness. The pain increases after she has been using a keyboard for several hours. She also experiences some pain in her forearm. She often needs to "shake out" her left hand when she awakens in the morning to get rid of the numbness. For the past 6 months she has also noticed some difficulty climbing stairs and she occasionally trips over curbs. She believes these symptoms have been gradually worsening. She is otherwise healthy and takes no medications other than etanercept. She neither smokes nor consumes alcohol.

She eats a normal diet. She has no family history of neurologic disease.

On examination, the patient is a well-developed, well-nourished middle-aged woman who appears healthy. She is afebrile, with BP 110/70 and pulse 72 and regular. The general physical examination is noteworthy only for mild to moderate joint deformities in the interphalangeal joints of her hands, characteristic of RA, but without signs of active inflammation. The neurologic examination reveals normal mental status and cranial nerve function. On motor examination, her gait is mildly slow and she has slight circumduction of both legs. She is able to walk on her toes but has difficulty walking on her heels. Tandem gait is normal. Muscle tone is normal in the upper extremities but mildly spastic in both legs. Manual muscle testing is normal in the upper extremities. In her lower extremities, the hip flexors are 4+ bilaterally, as are the dorsiflexors of the feet. The knee flexors are 5-. The other leg muscles are normal. Coordination testing is normal. Sensory examination reveals normal pinprick and light touch sensation throughout. Proprioception is normal, but she has moderately diminished vibratory sensation in her toes bilaterally. Deep tendon reflexes are hyperactive in the upper and lower extremities, with a few beats of ankle clonus bilaterally. Plantar responses are extensor bilaterally.

What do you do now?

The predominant feature of this woman's neurologic syndrome is a spastic paraparesis, and this warrants an expedited evaluation. Most important is MRI of the spinal cord in both the cervical and thoracic regions because this patient's examination does not provide a clear indication of the potential level of involvement. This is necessary to determine whether a compressive myelopathy is present, and the MRI may also show intrinsic lesions of the spinal cord to suggest an inflammatory/demyelinating process. Depending on the findings of the spinal cord imaging, additional imaging of the brain might be warranted if multiple sclerosis is a possibility. The signs of lateral column (spastic paraparesis) and dorsal column (impaired vibratory sensation) suggest the possibility of subacute combined degeneration, so vitamin B12 and methylmalonic acid levels should be determined. Though uncommon in this situation, serologic evidence for syphilis should also be sought. In some circumstances, CSF examination might be indicated.

RA is a systemic inflammatory disease that is characterized principally by a polyarthritis characterized by synovial inflammation, which can lead to destruction of cartilage and bone erosion. Although any synovial joint can be involved, most typical is inflammation and deformity of the proximal interphalangeal and metacarpophalangeal joints of the hands, often in a symmetric pattern.

RA can be associated with a number of neurologic complications. Most pertinent to this case is that of atlantoaxial subluxation, which can result in compression of the high cervical spinal cord. The rheumatoid inflammatory process leads to synovial proliferation, called *pannus*, which can damage adjacent ligaments, cartilage, and bones. If this involves the atlantoaxial joint, atlantoaxial subluxation may occur, which may result in compressive myelopathy. When mild, the subluxation is often asymptomatic. Early symptoms include neck pain and occipital headache. As the compression progresses, symptoms may include painless sensory loss in the hands and a mild spastic para- or quadriparesis. Although conservative management is appropriate for patients with no or mild symptoms, the presence of myelopathy warrants surgical intervention to stabilize the spine.

Other cervical spine abnormalities may also be associated with RA. Because of rheumatoid destruction of the articular facets (lateral masses) of the C2 vertebra, basilar invagination, also known as atlantoaxial impaction, may occur. This may cause lower cranial neuropathies and/or dysfunction of the pons or medulla. Usually developing later in the course of RA and less frequently, subaxial subluxation may also occur. Rheumatoid involvement of the meninges can occur but is rather uncommon. When it does occur, a pachymeningitis (i.e., dural involvement) is typical. However, inflammation of the leptomeninges may also be seen, either in combination with or independent of the dural process. Rheumatoid meningitis may elicit the typical symptoms and signs of meningeal irritation such as headache and stiff neck but may also be associated with seizures, cranial nerve involvement, and other focal abnormalities. Optimal therapy is uncertain and has included corticosteroids as well as many of the immunomodulating or immunosuppressive strategies that have been otherwise employed for the treatment of RA.

In the peripheral nervous system, a variety of neuropathies have been associated with RA. However, most typical are compressive neuropathies, which result from rheumatoid tenosynovitis or joint deformities. Probably the most common of these is carpal tunnel syndrome, resulting from compression of the medial nerve at the wrist. The patient described in this vignette, in addition to having an atlantoaxial subluxation resulting in the symptoms and signs of cervical myelopathy, also has left carpal tunnel syndrome. She manifests typical symptoms, which include pain radiating into the thumb, index, middle, and sometimes ring fingers (but sparing the pinky) and often pain in the forearm. The pain and numbness may awaken the patient from sleep and the numbness is often more prominent upon awakening in the morning. Symptoms may be aggravated by repetitive tasks involving the wrist. When severe, carpal tunnel syndrome may also result in motor weakness in the hand muscles innervated by the median nerve. Less common neuropathic syndromes in RA include mononeuritis multiplex or a distal symmetric, mainly sensory, polyneuropathy. The pathology in these cases, even in the latter presentation, is typically that of a necrotizing vasculitis.

A variety of medications are used to treat RA and many of these have been associated, on occasion, with neurologic complications. Particularly germane to the patient described here is the occurrence of CNS demyelinating events with the use of tumor necrosis factor-α (TNF-α) inhibitors. Etanercept had been most frequently associated with this complication, but other TNF-α inhibitors, including infliximab and adalimumab, have also been implicated. Low-dose oral methotrexate is widely used for treatment of RA. Only rarely has this been associated with a severe leukoencephalopathy, which is much more commonly encountered with intravenous or intrathecal methotrexate therapy, usually administered for the treatment of malignancy. The anti-B-cell monoclonal antibody rituximab, which is approved for treatment of moderate or severe refractory RA, has been rarely associated with the development of progressive multifocal leukoencephalopathy. Leflunomide, which inhibits T-lymphocyte proliferation, has occasionally resulted in the development of a distal polyneuropathy, either pure sensory or sensorimotor in nature. Finally, while seldom used today, the older disease-modifying antirheumatic agents, gold and D-penicillamine, have been associated with neuropathy and drug-induced autoimmune myasthenia gravis, respectively.

KEY POINTS TO REMEMBER

- Atlantoaxial subluxation is a very important neurologic complication of RA that my result in compressive myelopathy.
- Rheumatoid meningitis is uncommon but tends to involve the dura when it does occur.
- A variety of peripheral neuropathies are associated with RA, but compressive neuropathies are most common.
- A variety of medications are used to treat RA, and many of these have been associated, on occasion, with neurologic complications

---

Further Reading

Agarwal AK, Peppelman WC Jr, Kraus DR, Eisenbeis CH Jr. The cervical spine in rheumatoid arthritis. *BMJ* 1993; 306(6870):79-80.

Kim DH, Hilibrand AS. Rheumatoid arthritis in the cervical spine. *J Am Acad Orthop Surg* 2005; 13(7):463-474.

Lewis SL. Neurologic complications of Sjogren syndrome and rheumatoid arthritis. *Continuum* 2008; 14(1):120-144.

Thomas CW Jr, Weinshenker BG, Sandborn WJ. Demyelination during anti-tumor necrosis factor alpha therapy with infliximab for Crohn's disease. *Inflamm Bowel Dis* 2004; 10(1):28-31.

13 Neuro-Behçet's Disease

A 42-year-old man with a past medical history of oral and genital herpes presents to the emergency room with 3 days of double vision and slurred speech. He now reports his left face is numb and tingling, and his walking is becoming increasingly unsteady. His only medications are valacyclovir and ibuprofen for occasional arthritic pain in his knees. Despite chronic valacyclovir, he continues to have outbreaks of ulcers two or three times yearly. On neurologic examination, he has a left sixth nerve palsy, diminished sensation to pain and temperature involving the left face, mild flattening of the left nasolabial fold, and labial dysarthria. His gait is slightly wide-based and mildly unsteady, with occasional listing to the left. An MRI of the brain discloses a left pontine T2/FLAIR hyperintense lesion with gadolinium enhancement. He is admitted to the hospital for further testing. A lumbar puncture demonstrates a lymphocytic pleocytosis of 12 cells with moderately elevated protein. Viral cultures, specifically PCR for herpesviridae and JC virus, as well as AFB smears, PCR for *Treponema whipplei*, VDRL, Lyme antibodies, CSF ACE level and cytology are negative. Oligoclonal bands are absent and IgG synthesis and index are normal. Serum HIV testing is negative. Prior to initiation of IV corticosteroids, a dermatologist performs a Tzanck smear of an actively inflamed genital lesion, and the results, along with viral culture, are negative for herpes simplex-2 virus. His neurologic symptoms gradually improve with 5 days of IV methylprednisolone. The determination that his orogenital ulcerations are non-herpetic prompts consideration of a brain stem lesion secondary to neurologic sequelae of BehÁet's disease. A pathergy test is performed on his right forearm and demonstrates a positive reaction approximately 48 hours after pinprick. A serum HLA-B51 test is positive.

What do you do now?

In this case, the occurrence of a brain stem inflammatory syndrome in a patient with a history of recurrent non-herpetic orogenital ulcerations should raise suspicion for neuro-Behçet's disease, in addition to a differential diagnosis that includes infectious, inflammatory, demyelinating, granulomatous, and neoplastic processes. A thorough evaluation including MRI of the brain with and without gadolinium contrast, as well as CSF analysis for viral and bacterial infections such as herpes simplex 2, Lyme, tuberculosis, syphilis, and Whipple's disease, should be obtained. CSF determination of, oligoclonal bands, IgG synthesis and index for demyelinating disease, ACE level for neurosarcoidosis, and cytology for lymphoma should be pursued to exclude such alternative possible etiologies for an inflammatory brain stem lesion.

Behçet's disease is a multisystemic, inflammatory disorder first described by Hippocrates and later characterized by Hulusi Behçet in 1937. There is no specific laboratory test for Behçet's disease. Diagnosis rests primarily on the characteristic clinical signs and symptoms of recurrent, orogenital mucocutaneous ulcerations, uveitis, and skin lesions. Arthritic, gastrointestinal, and neurologic symptoms can also occur, the last in approximately 10% to 20% of cases. The disease is more common in populations originating along the ancient "silk route" in the Middle and Far Eastern regions.

Several diagnostic criteria have been proposed for Behçet's disease over the years. The most recently adopted international criteria were published in 1990 and require the following: presence of recurrent oral aphthous ulcers (at least three times annually) in addition to two of the following four requisites and the absence of other systemic diseases:

- Recurrent genital aphthous ulcers
- Eye lesions (anterior or posterior uveitis or retinal vasculitis)
- Skin lesions (erythema nodosum, pseudo-vasculitis, papulopustular lesions, acneiform nodules)
- A positive pathergy test (development of a papule 2 mm or more in size within 24 to 48 hours after oblique insertion of a 20- to 25-gauge needle 5 mm into the skin, generally performed on the forearm)

This patient has a history of recurrent oral and genital ulcers at the aforementioned frequency and a positive pathergy test; therefore, in the absence of any other systemic disease, he meets the criteria for a diagnosis of Behçet's disease.

The pathophysiology of Behçet's disease involves an inflammatory, probably vasculitic, state, which distinctly can involve arteries of all sizes. Laboratory testing generally demonstrates nonspecific evidence of inflammation—for example, elevated white blood cell count, erythrocyte sedimentation rate, and C-reactive protein. HLA-B51 has been correlated with disease in affected individuals from high-prevalence areas.

Neurologic disease is more common in men than women and generally manifests roughly 5 years after the diagnosis of non-neurologic symptoms, although rarely neurologic involvement can predate or occur in isolation of systemic symptomatology. Various neurologic symptoms have been described, ranging from aseptic meningoencephalitis, commonly involving the brain stem, to vasculitis, neuropsychiatric impairment, focal parenchymal lesions, and arterial and venous sinus thromboses. MRI of the brain and spinal cord can demonstrate focal parenchymal lesions typically involving the brain stem, periventricular white matter, corticospinal tracts, basal ganglia, spinal cord, and, rarely, cerebellum. Peripheral neuropathy is uncommon. Potential complications of neuro-Behçet's vasculitis include stroke, dissection, aneurysm, and subarachnoid hemorrhage. CSF profiles generally disclose a lymphocytic pleocytosis with elevated protein, and in the setting of venous sinus thrombosis, an elevated CSF opening pressure. Pathologic specimens from nervous system tissue demonstrate inflammatory infiltrates with perivenular lymphocytic cuffing, gliosis, neuronal loss and necrosis.

The mainstay of treatment for Behçet's disease involves courses of low- to high-dose oral and IV corticosteroids, although this therapeutic approach has been subject to few randomized controlled trials. Treatment is dictated typically by specific organ system involvement and severity of disease. Acute neurologic disease is generally treated with high doses of IV corticosteroids followed by an oral steroid taper, with consideration of initiation of maintenance steroid-sparing immunosuppressants such as azathioprine, methotrexate, mycophenolate mofetil, cyclophosphamide, or cyclosporine, to prevent further attacks. CNS parenchymal lesions and elevated CSF protein have been correlated with a poor prognosis; therefore, this patient should be started on a maintenance therapy. Venous sinus thromboses secondary to Behçet's disease are generally treated with standard anticoagulation therapy and continuation of maintenance immunosuppression. Ongoing multidisciplinary surveillance from a team including subspecialists from neurology, rheumatology, ophthalmology, and dermatology is strongly recommended.

KEY POINTS TO REMEMBER

- Neurologic involvement in Behçet's disease occurs in approximately 10% to 20% of patients, typically 5 years after the onset of non-neurologic disease.
- Neuro-Behçet's disease can involve aseptic meningoencephalitis, vasculitis, neuropsychiatric impairment, focal brain parenchymal lesions, and arterial and venous sinus thrombosis.
- The mainstay of therapy in neuro-Behçet's disease is corticosteroids and immunosuppressant agents.

Further Reading

Akman-Demir G, Serdaroglu P, Tasci B. Clinical patterns of neurological involvement in BehÁet's disease. *Jpn J Ophthalmol* 2006; 50:256.

Benamour S, Naji T, Alaoui FZ, et al. Neurological involvement in BehÁet's disease. 154 cases from a cohort of 925 patients and review of the literature. *Rev Neurol (Paris)* 2006; 162:1084.

Kidd D, Steuer A, Denman AM, et al. Neurological complications in BehÁet's syndrome. *Brain* 1999; 122(Pt 11):2183.

14 Sjögren's Syndrome

A 35-year-old woman presents with a chief complaint of numbness and tingling of her feet and unsteadiness walking for the past two months. Two years ago she developed numbness of the left side of her face, which has persisted. She has never had any visual symptoms, but does note that her eyes often feel uncomfortable, as if there is something gritty present. She denies any history of vertigo, but she does report that she often feels lightheaded, especially when she gets out of bed. On two such occasions she felt as if she were going to pass out, so she sat back down until the sensation passed in a few minutes. She has otherwise been healthy with no other significant past medical or surgical history. In her marketing job she has to give frequent oral presentations. She notes that she frequently has to take sips of water during these occasions, which she has attributed to mild anxiety. A maternal grandmother was diagnosed with multiple sclerosis. The patient drinks a glass or two of wine approximately twice a week. She does not use tobacco and denies any use of recreational drugs. The review of systems is otherwise negative. She denies any urinary or bowel symptoms. She has not had any joint pain, stiffness, or swelling. She has not noticed any skin rashes.

On physical examination, she is a well-developed, well-nourished woman in no distress. Her BP is 110/70 supine and falls to 80/50 after 3 minutes of standing. The resting pulse was 76 and regular, rising to 80 after standing. The remainder of the general physical examination was unremarkable. On neurologic examination, the mental status was normal. Cranial nerve examination revealed the pupils to be equal and 3 mm in diameter. Both pupils constricted very sluggishly to light, but briskly when she was asked to fixate on a near object. Extraocular movements were full with no nystagmus. Facial sensation was diminished to pinprick in the left V2-3 distribution. The rest of the cranial nerve examination was normal. Motor examination revealed normal strength and tone throughout. The gait was wide-based and unsteady. Finger-to-nose testing, rapid alternating movements, and heel-knee-shin tests were performed normally. She had a positive Romberg sign. Sensory examination revealed normal pinprick and light touch. However, vibratory sensation was absent in the lower extremities and moderately impaired in the upper extremities. She had significant impairment of joint position sense at the toes and ankles and could not detect small excursions of movement in her fingers. Deep tendon reflexes were unobtainable.

The patient's primary care physician suspected that she had multiple sclerosis and ordered an MRI of the brain with and without administration of gadolinium. The MRI showed two 3-mm T2 hyperintense lesions in the peripheral subcortical white matter. He also ordered a battery of laboratory investigations, including complete blood count, chemistries, and erythrocyte sedimentation rate, which were normal. Antibody testing for Lyme disease was negative. He then referred the patient for neurologic consultation.

What do you do now?

This patient has a clinical syndrome strongly suggestive of primary Sjögren's syndrome. The gritty sensation in her eyes and the need to drink water during her oral presentations imply the presence of the sicca syndrome, consisting of dry eyes and dry mouth. In addition, she has evidence of involvement of the peripheral nervous system, the most common neurologic manifestations of Sjögren's.

Serologic studies for the presence of the antibodies against the ribonucleoprotein complexes Ro (SSA) and LA (SSB) should be performed. These antibodies are found in approximately 60% of cases of Sjögren's, although their presence is not specific to the disorder. Documentation of the presence of xerophthalmia can be obtained by performing the Schirmer test to measure tear production. More definitive diagnosis depends on the finding of lymphocytic infiltration of minor salivary glands (lip biopsy).

A wide variety of peripheral neuropathic manifestations occur in Sjögren's. Most frequent is sensory ataxia, which typically begins with distal paresthesias, which then may spread proximally. This is followed by gait ataxia and, in severe cases, significant proprioceptive abnormalities in the hands as well. Pseudo-athetoid movements of the fingers may occur. This patient demonstrates evidence for this type of neuropathy by the findings of impaired vibratory and proprioceptive sense, gait ataxia, positive Romberg sign, and areflexia. The clinical manifestations result from lymphocytic infiltration of the dorsal root ganglia; thus, the syndrome is actually a sensory neuronopathy. Electrodiagnostic studies will show reduced or absent sensory nerve action potentials.

Autonomic neuropathy may exist by itself in Sjögren's patients, or it may accompany sensory ataxia. This patient demonstrated Adie's tonic pupil, in which usually one pupil is large and constricts very sluggishly to light but briskly to the near reflex. In addition, she has evidence for orthostatic hypotension. Another type of peripheral neuropathy, that involving the trigeminal nerve, is also common, and this patient manifests impairment of pinprick sensation on the face. Other types of peripheral neuropathy encountered in Sjögren's include painful sensory neuropathy without ataxia, mononeuritis multiplex, multiple cranial neuropathies, and radiculoneuropathy. The mononeuritis multiplex, and possibly the multiple cranial neuropathies, is likely due to vasculitis, which may be demonstrated on sural nerve biopsy.

Treatment of the various forms of neuropathy has been difficult, and judgment of the effectiveness of therapy is clouded by the fact that some patients stabilize or improve spontaneously. Particularly regarding the sensory ataxia, most reports have found that only a relatively small minority of patients appear to respond to corticosteroids, and treatment with intravenous immunoglobulin has also yielded inconsistent results.

Less common than peripheral nerve manifestations, CNS involvement can occur. In some patients, a syndrome mimicking multiple sclerosis can occur and the brain MRI may show multiple lesions characteristic of that disorder. This patient, however, lacked evidence for CNS involvement and had only a couple of small, nonspecific T2 hyperintense lesions on brain MRI. The occurrence of neuromyelitis optica (see Chapter 5) is rather common in the presence of Sjögren's syndrome but most likely represents the coexistence of two autoimmune disorders.

KEY POINTS TO REMEMBER

- The sicca syndrome (xerophthalmia and xerostomia) is common in Sjögren's syndrome. Pathologic confirmation can be obtained by a biopsy of a minor salivary gland.
- The characteristic antibodies, anti-RO (SSA) and anti-LA (SSB), are present in approximately 60% of patients, but their presence is not specific for Sjögren's syndrome.
- A variety of peripheral neuropathies occur in Sjögren's and are the most typical neurologic manifestations.
- CNS involvement may occur and sometimes mimics multiple sclerosis.

Further Reading

Birnbaum J. Peripheral nervous system manifestations of Sjögren syndrome: clinical patterns, diagnostic paradigms, etiopathogenesis, and therapeutic strategies. *Neurologist* 2010; 16(5):287-297.

Chai J, Logigian EL. Neurological manifestations of primary Sjögren's syndrome. *Curr Opin Neurol* 2010; 23(5):509-513.

Mellgren SI, Goransson LG, Omdal R. Primary Sjögren's syndrome-associated neuropathy. *Can J Neurol Sci* 2007; 34(3):280-287.

Segal B, Carpenter A, Walk D. Involvement of nervous system pathways in primary Sjögren's syndrome. *Rheum Dis Clin North Am.* 2008; 34(4):885-906.

15   Neurosarcoidosis

A 40-year-old African-American man presented for neurologic consultation because on the previous day he had noticed drooping of the right side of his mouth and difficulty closing his right eye. He reported that he had been experiencing nearly continuous headache over the past 3 weeks and excessive fatigue, but he attributed these symptoms to increased stress at his job as a retail sales manager. He denied any other current or prior neurologic symptoms. He denied any history of visual disturbance or other ophthalmologic problems. He denies recent fever.

Past medical history was entirely unremarkable. His only medication has been over-the-counter ibuprofen 400 mg twice daily for his recent headaches.

He is married. He drinks approximately four beers weekly but denies other alcohol use. He does not use tobacco but admits to smoking marijuana occasionally. He denies other illicit drug use. He was born in and has always lived in North Carolina. He denies any recent travel.

His mother has type 2 diabetes mellitus. His father, who was a heavy smoker, died of lung cancer at age 60.

Two siblings are healthy. The patient has two daughters, age 12 and 9, who are well.

Review of systems is negative except that the patient reports some recent dyspnea on exertion. He has had difficulty running up and down the court in his regular weekly basketball game and also has noticed some shortness of breath after climbing several flights of stairs during the past few weeks.

Physical examination reveals a well-developed, well-nourished African-American man who appears comfortable. He is afebrile. Blood pressure is 125/75; pulse 72 regular; respiratory rate 12. There is neck stiffness when the neck is flexed and a positive Brudzinski sign is noted. Bilateral axillary lymphadenopathy is noted. The remainder of the general physical examination is normal.

On neurologic examination, the mental status is normal. Cranial nerve examination reveals a moderately severe right facial nerve paresis of the peripheral type (i.e., includes weakness of eye closure and brow wrinkling in addition to lower face weakness). The remainder of the cranial nerve examination is normal, including visual acuity and funduscopic examination. Examination of the motor and sensory systems and tests of coordination are normal. Deep tendon reflexes are 2+ and symmetric throughout and the plantar responses are flexor.

What do you do now?

Y ou should have a strong suspicion for the possibility of neurosarcoidosis in this patient. The subacute persistent headache accompanied by signs on physical examination of meningeal irritation suggests a subacute or chronic form of meningitis. This and peripheral facial palsy are among the most frequent neurologic manifestations of sarcoidosis. These neurologic findings, along with the history of dyspnea on exertion and the finding on physical examination of lymphadenopathy, should place sarcoidosis at the top of the differential diagnosis.

Sarcoidosis is a multisystem inflammatory disorder of unknown etiology, characterized pathologically by the presence of noncaseating granulomas and multinucleated giant cells. For unknown reasons, the disorder tends to be more common among African Americans and, in the United States, seems to occur more frequently in the mid-Atlantic states. Among the most common systemic manifestations are pulmonary involvement, lymphadenopathy, and skin lesions. A definite diagnosis can be made only by biopsy of an affected organ.

Involvement of the central or peripheral nervous system occurs in approximately 5% of people with sarcoidosis. The neurologic manifestations can coexist with systemic involvement or can occur alone. In a review of 83 patients from the Mayo Clinic (cited in Aksamit A 2008).

Thirty seven percent had been diagnosed with systemic sarcoidosis at least 6 months before the neurologic manifestations. In 28%, the neurologic symptoms were the initial presentation of the disorder, but on evaluation evidence of other systemic involvement was found. In the remaining 35% of patients only CNS sarcoidosis was found, confirmed by nervous tissue biopsy. Because of the tertiary referral population of the Mayo Clinic, it is possible that this figure for isolated neurologic involvement is higher than would be seen in other samples (Figs. 15-1 and 15-2).

Chronic meningitis with headache, often accompanied by encephalopathy or cranial nerve palsy, is the most frequent neurologic presentation, occurring in 78% of patients in the Mayo Clinic review. Suspicion of meningitis dictates performance of a lumbar puncture for definitive demonstration of inflammation, and the procedure should be performed in this patient. In sarcoidosis, characteristic CSF findings include a moderate lymphocytic pleocytosis and mild to moderate protein elevation. The CSF glucose level is usually normal, but occasionally hypoglycorrhachia is found.

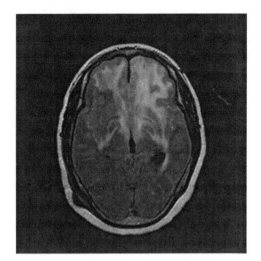

FIGURE 15-1

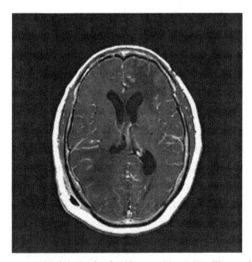

FIGURES 15-1 and 15-2   MRI of the brain of a 40-year-old woman with sarcoidosis presenting with headache, bitemporal field defects, disinhibition, hyperphagia, and diabetes insipidus demonstrates extensive infiltrative process involving the sella and suprasellar regions, bilateral orbitofrontal lobes (Fig. 15-1) with surrounding vasogenic edema in the frontal and parietal lobes as well as diffuse leptomeningeal thickening and enhancement (Fig. 15-2). Brain biopsy demonstrated noncaseating granulomas, consistent with neurosarcoidosis.

It is important to obtain a serum glucose level at the same time that the CSF glucose level is determined.

The neurologic manifestations of sarcoidosis are protean, but cranial neuropathies are the next most common feature. Involvement of the facial nerve is particularly frequent, but involvement of the optic nerve or the vestibulocochlear nerve is common. Other cranial nerves are less commonly involved.

Another fairly common neurologic syndrome in sarcoidosis is myelopathy, with patients typically presenting with paraparesis. In some patients involvement of the conus medullaris, characterized by prominent bladder and bowel symptoms, is evident. Another area of CNS involvement that characterizes neurosarcoidosis is the hypothalamus or pituitary area. Inflammation in this region may cause diabetes insipidus, other hypothalamic endocrinologic dysfunction, or symptoms related to involvement of the optic chiasm (Aksamit, 2008).

KEY POINTS TO REMEMBER

- Sarcoidosis is a multisystem inflammatory disorder of unknown etiology, characterized pathologically by the presence of noncaseating granulomas and multinucleated giant cells.
- Chronic meningitis with headache, often accompanied by encephalopathy or cranial nerve palsy, is the most frequent neurologic presentation of sarcoidosis.
- Involvement of the facial nerve is particularly frequent, but involvement of the optic nerve or the vestibulocochlear nerve is common.
- Inflammation in the region of the pituitary gland or hypothalamus may cause diabetes insipidus, other hypothalamic endocrinologic dysfunction, or symptoms related to involvement of the optic chiasm.

Further Reading
Aksamit A. Neurosarcoidosis. *Continuum: Lifelong Learning in Neurology* 2008; 14(1):181-196.

Hoitsma E, Drent M, Sharma OP. A pragmatic approach to diagnosing and treating neurosarcoidosis in the 21st century. *Curr Opin Pulm Med* 2010; 16(5):472-479.

Terushkin V, Stern BJ, Judson MA, et al. Neurosarcoidosis: presentations and management. *Neurologist* 2010; 16(1):2-15.

Vargas DL, Stern BJ. Neurosarcoidosis: diagnosis and management. *Semin Respir Crit Care Med* 2010; 31(4):419-427.

16   Susac's Syndrome

A 20-year-old woman with an unremarkable past medical history presents to the emergency room with 3 days of severe headaches and ringing in her ears. Her sister reports that she has appeared confused and forgetful lately, leaving her wallet at the grocery store twice and missing their weekly yoga class. She has also expressed worry than someone is going to break into her home. She complains of episodic blurry vision, trouble hearing from her left ear, and unsteady gait. She denies any fever or recent infections or vaccinations. She denies tobacco or alcohol use and has no history of illicit drug use. She is an art history student and traveled to Barcelona with friends 3 months ago to study painting. On examination, her vital signs are normal. General examination is unremarkable. On neurologic examination, she is somnolent but arousable. She is oriented to self and place but does not know the date. Her affect is flattened and inattentive. Speech is clear and fluent. She has trouble following simple commands and she remembers only one of three items at 5 minutes. Cranial nerve examination demonstrates normal fundi bilaterally, visual acuity of 20/50 bilaterally, and diminished hearing in her left ear. Motor examination demonstrates full power throughout with brisk symmetric reflexes and bilateral extensor plantar responses. Sensory examination is normal to all modalities. Coordination testing reveals dysmetria with right finger-to-nose testing and bilaterally dystaxic heel-knee-shin testing. Her gait is wide-based and ataxic. She can heel and toe walk but tandem walking is moderately impaired. A CT scan of the head demonstrates tiny hypodense foci throughout the cerebral hemispheres. MRI of the brain reveals multiple tiny diffusion restricted T2/FLAIR hyperintense white matter lesions, some of which enhance after gadolinium administration. Several lesions involve the central portion of the corpus callosum demonstrating a moth-eaten appearance. A lumbar puncture discloses a lymphocytic pleocytosis with 18 white cells, 87% lymphocytes, 2 red blood cells, and elevated protein of 86. The patient is started on empiric acyclovir until CSF HSV-1/2, CMV, and EBV PCR results come back normal. Additional CSF studies for VDRL, Lyme, and varicella zoster virus are negative. CSF oligoclonal bands are positive and cytology is benign. Laboratory studies including complete blood count, chemistries, vitamin B12, HIV, and thyroid function tests are normal, and an MRI of the cervicothoracic spine is unremarkable. Neuro-ophthalmologic examination demonstrates bilateral branched retinal artery occlusions (BRAOs).

What do you do now?

Acute to subacute alteration in mental status in the presence of vision and hearing loss, ataxia and bilaterally extensor plantar responses, should prompt an evaluation for CNS pathology. Important initial considerations include aseptic meningitides, demyelinating disease such as acute disseminated encephalomyelitis, toxic metabolic encephalopathies, and CNS vasculitides, followed by less common entities such as neoplastic or paraneoplastic encephalitides.

In the presence of multiple T2 hyperintense white matter lesions, the possibility of acute disseminated encephalomyelitis (ADEM) or a first episode of multiple sclerosis (MS) should be strongly considered, with the presence of encephalopathy favoring the former. CSF studies demonstrating a lymphocytic pleocytosis and elevated protein would be compatible with ADEM or MS. Oligoclonal bands are uncommon in ADEM but have been reported. It is always important when attempting to gauge the likelihood of demyelinating disease versus mimicking etiologies to rigorously assess the patient's history and examination to determine whether an alternative explanation may better explain the symptomatology (Fig. 16-1).

In this case, the patient's encephalopathy was accompanied by significant vision and hearing loss. In this clinical setting, Susac's syndrome, or

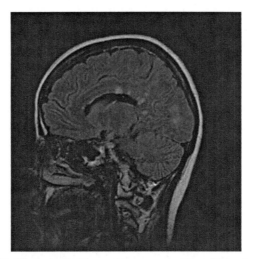

FIGURE 16-1 MRI of the brain of a 31-year-old woman presenting with headache, bilateral hearing loss, encephalopathy, and blurry vision demonstrates the pathognomonic T2/FLAIR central callosal "snowball" and spoke lesions.

retinocochleocerebral encephalopathy, should be strongly considered with its classical triad of altered mental status, vision impairment involving BRAOs, and hearing loss. Susac's affects women more often than men. Onset is generally between the ages of 20 to 40, but SS has been reported with an age range extending from 7 to 72 years old. The complete triad of symptoms may not always be present at the outset, lowering diagnostic suspicion and making early diagnosis difficult. Headache, frequently migrainous, generally accompanies the encephalopathy and can best be attributed to leptomeningeal involvement. Headaches can predate the presentation by several months. Encephalopathy typically features neuropsychiatric manifestations, such as depression and paranoia, as well as confusion and memory impairment.

MRI findings are frequently confused with demyelinating disease with white matter hyperintensities involving the supra- and infratentorial regions; however, a distinct imaging finding present in this patient which is atypical for MS and characteristic of Susac's is evidence of central corpus callosal lesions, which are considered essentially pathognomonic for SS. Central callosal lesions appear as rounded T2 hyperintensities ("snowballs") that evolve into T1 hypointense regions ("holes"), similar to the black holes described in chronic demyelinating lesions. In comparison to MS, the callosal–septal interface is spared. Interestingly, when encephalopathy is present, callosal lesions appear to be uniformly present. A sagittal T2/FLAIR sequence is critical for ideal visualization of these lesions and must be requested by the treating clinician, as it is not a routine part of MRI protocols. Also, deep gray matter lesions, as well as leptomeningeal involvement, have been noted in 70% and 33% of cases respectively. These lesions may enhance after gadolinium administration and further distinguish Susac's from MS. In patients with long tract findings, microinfarcts involving the internal capsule have been demonstrated in a configuration described as a "string of pearls," best illustrated by diffusion-weighted imaging sequences. CSF studies generally demonstrate a lymphocytic pleocytosis and elevated protein, warranting further evaluation for possible infectious and inflammatory etiologies. Oligoclonal bands are generally absent.

A very important diagnostic evaluation in suspected Susac's cases is a detailed neuro-ophthalmologic examination looking for BRAOs, which can be best demonstrated by retinal fluoroscein angiography. BRAOs lead to segmental loss in the visual fields of one or both eyes, either subtle or severe. If initial fluoroscein angiography is normal, repeat testing should be considered in a suspicious clinical context. In addition to ophthalmologic evaluation, audiometry is important to demonstrate cochlear sensorineural hearing loss, which is usually bilateral and can lead to permanent deafness. The hearing loss involves low- to medium-range frequencies, causing poor speech discrimination, which is attributed anatomically to microinfarcts of the apical cochlea. Associated vestibular symptoms have been described, ranging from vertigo and dystaxia to unsteady gait, secondary to either central or peripheral involvement.

The clinical course of Susac's is generally monophasic but with fluctuating attacks. It demonstrates a self-limited course involving one or more of the components of the triad, with activity occurring for periods of time from 2 months to a decade, with a mean duration of 2 years. Residual cognitive, vision, and hearing loss can occur; therefore, early diagnosis and treatment is strongly recommended. Late recurrence after remission has been reported in only a single case.

The etiology of Susac's syndrome is unknown, but immunologic and post-infectious mechanisms causing multiple microinfarcts have been implicated by pathologic studies and therapeutic response to immunosuppressant therapy. High-dose corticosteroids are the mainstay of treatment, but alternative immunosuppressant regimens, including cyclophosphamide, intravenous immunoglobulin, plasma exchange, and recently rituximab, have been reported anecdotally, in addition to antiplatelet therapy.

KEY POINTS TO REMEMBER

- Susac's syndrome, or retinocochleocerebral vasculopathy, involves the triad of encephalopathy, vision loss with multiple BRAOs, and hearing loss.
- Corpus callosal lesions typically involve the central fibers and appear to be pathognomonic for the disorder.
- Hearing loss in Susac's is usually acute, bilateral, albeit asymmetric, and sensorineural.
- There is no proven therapy for Susac's, but the suspicion of an autoimmune etiology has informed empiric treatment with corticosteroids and various immunosuppressant regimens with variable results.

Further Reading

Gross M, Eliashar R. Update on Susac's syndrome. *Curr Opin Neurol* 2005; 18:311-314.

Lian K, Siripurapu R, Yeung R, et al. Susac's syndrome. *Can J Neurol Sci* 2011; 38: 335-337.

Rennebohm R, Susac JO, Egan RA, Daroff RB. Susac's syndrome: update. *J Neurol Sci* 2010; 299:86-91.

17 Neuropsychiatric Systemic Lupus Erythematosus

A 25-year-old previously healthy woman was diagnosed with systemic lupus erythematosus (SLE) one year ago after she presented with malar rash and chest pain. She was found to have pericarditis and workup revealed 3+ proteinuria. Complete blood count was normal except for a platelet count of 75,000/mm³. Evaluation showed an antinuclear antibody (ANA) titer of 1:1,280 and the presence of anti-double-stranded DNA. She was treated initially with intravenous methylprednisolone and then tapering doses of oral corticosteroids. Her symptoms improved, with resolution of the pericarditis and reduction to trace proteinuria. She was maintained on low-dose oral prednisone (10 mg daily), as well as hydroxychloroquine, and remained well until she presented acutely with two generalized seizures on the day of admission. She was treated with intravenous diazepam (Valium) and fosphenytoin and had no further seizures, but on the day following admission she remained lethargic and confused. She was febrile to

101ºF. Urinalysis showed microscopic hematuria and 2+ proteinuria. Her serum creatinine was 2.8 mg/dL.

What do you do now?

SLE is a multiple-organ disorder that is diagnosed based on the presence of four or more of the following conditions:

1. Malar rash: Fixed erythema, flat or raised, over the malar eminences
2. Discoid rash: Erythematous circular raised patches with adherent keratotic scaling and follicular plugging; atrophic scarring may occur
3. Photosensitivity: Exposure to ultraviolet light causes rash
4. Oral ulcers: Includes oral and nasopharyngeal ulcers, observed by physician
5. Arthritis: Non-erosive arthritis of two or more peripheral joints, with tenderness, swelling, or effusion
6. Serositis: Pleuritis or pericarditis documented by ECG or rub or evidence of effusion
7. Renal disorder: Proteinuria >0.5 g/d or 3+, or cellular casts
8. Neurologic disorder: Seizures or psychosis without other causes
9. Hematologic disorder: Hemolytic anemia or leukopenia (<4,000/L) or lymphopenia (<1,500/L) or thrombocytopenia (<100,000/L) in the absence of offending drugs
10. Immunologic disorder: Anti-dsDNA, anti-Sm, and/or antiphospholipid
11. ANAs: An abnormal titer of ANA by immunofluorescence or an equivalent assay at any point in time in the absence of drugs known to induce ANAs

In this case, the criteria were originally satisfied by the presence of malar rash, serositis (pericarditis), renal disorder, thrombocytopenia, and the presence of ANA and anti-dsDNA. The mainstay of treatment for acute exacerbations of SLE is high-dose corticosteroids. At times this may need to be augmented with immunosuppressive agents such as cyclophosphamide or rituximab.

When a patient with SLE develops neurologic symptoms, the first question that must be asked is whether the episode is a direct consequence of the inflammatory disease; an indirect effect, such as a result of an affected organ outside the nervous system or an adverse event associated with treatment; or simply an unrelated event. When there are clinical signs of active inflammatory SLE, as evidenced by acute involvement outside the nervous system, a good possibility exists that an acute direct disease-related event is also occurring within the nervous system.

In this case, the occurrence of seizures, in and of themselves, should prompt a specific workup. However, the presence of an acute confusional state is particularly worrisome and may trigger additional investigation. The possibility of infection is always a serious concern in a patient with SLE, and meningoencephalitis or even brain abscess must be considered. The former may be present even in the absence of signs of meningeal irritation, especially in a patient on immunosuppressive agents, including corticosteroids. It is critical to perform a lumbar puncture in a patient such as this, although the clinician may wish first to perform an imaging study to rule out the relatively unlikely possibility of a space-occupying mass causing raised intracranial pressure. A CT scan is likely to be more quickly obtained, but ultimately an MRI might yield more specific diagnostic information. The CSF, in addition to routine studies, should be evaluated for unusual infections, such as tuberculosis or fungal infection. It is important for the clinician to recognize that the CSF in SLE patients may demonstrate a pleocytosis (usually 20 to 100 cells/µL), mild protein elevation, and even mildly reduced glucose even in the absence of infection.

An electroencephalogram (EEG) must be obtained urgently in a patient such as this. In a patient with a confusional state following clinically evident seizures, it is important to rule out the possibility of continuing, clinically inapparent seizures, a situation known as nonconvulsive status epilepticus.

In SLE, actual neurologic events are frequently ischemic rather than inflammatory. Thrombotic events are common as a direct manifestation of the disease but may also occur as a consequence of the anticardiolipin antibody syndrome that may be associated with SLE, or as a secondary cardioembolic event related to involvement of the heart. For example, so-called Libman-Sacks (i.e., noninfectious) endocarditis may occur.

If an ischemic event is identified, the management is often similar to that in patients without SLE. Inquiry about other vascular risk factors, including smoking, hypertension, diabetes mellitus, and hyperlipidemia, should be made and abnormalities treated appropriately. Long-term antiplatelet therapy will often be warranted. In patients with persistently elevated antiphospholipid antibodies, oral anticoagulation is usually indicated.

Occasionally patients will have intracerebral or subarachnoid hemorrhage. This may be precipitated by thrombocytopenia, though platelet counts below 50,000/mm^3 or even lower are generally necessary to induce bleeding. Therefore, bleeding is unlikely to have occurred in this particular patient.

In general, three types of risk factors have been associated with an increased frequency of neuropsychiatric events in SLE. The first is evidence of an active inflammatory state, as reflected by involvement of major organs, increased disease severity scores, serologic signs of immunoreactivity, and the use of high doses of corticosteroids or other immunosuppressive drugs. The second risk factor is the occurrence of prior neuropsychiatric SLE events, and the third is the presence of the antiphospholipid antibody syndrome, indicated by the finding of persistent moderate to high levels of anticardiolipin antibody or lupus anticoagulant positivity. Overall, recent reports suggest a cumulative incidence of neuropsychiatric SLE of 30% to 40%. Many of these manifestations occur at the onset of the disease or within a short time thereafter.

Common neuropsychiatric events, in addition to seizures and vascular events, include depression, anxiety, and headaches. However, it is unclear whether these are actually direct consequences of the disease pathology or, rather, secondary or coincidental events. Specific SLE manifestations that are regarded as uncommon (occurring in 1% to 5% of affected patients) include psychosis, polyneuropathy, and myelopathy, in addition to an acute confusional state, as described in this patient.

A large variety of other neuropsychiatric SLE syndromes may rarely (i.e., in <1% of patients) occur. These may include demyelinating syndromes of the CNS or the peripheral nervous system (Guillain-Barré syndrome), cranial or peripheral neuropathy (either single or multiplex), autonomic disorders, aseptic meningitis, plexopathy, or even myasthenia gravis. Brain imaging in lupus patients often shows T2 hyperintense lesions that are relatively nonspecific.

The treatment of neuropsychiatric SLE is not based on randomized, placebo-controlled, blinded studies. Nonetheless, when neuropsychiatric manifestations are thought to be on an immunologic or inflammatory basis, the use of corticosteroids alone or in combination with immunosuppressive agents such as azathioprine or cyclophosphamide is generally recommended.

In severe cases that are unresponsive to the more commonly used immunosuppressive regimens, plasmapheresis, IVIg, and recently rituximab, a monoclonal antibody directed against the B-cell antigen CD20, have been used.

> **KEY POINTS TO REMEMBER**
>
> - SLE is a multiple-organ disorder that is diagnosed based on the presence of four or more conditions from a list of possibilities that include skin manifestations, arthritis, serositis, and neurologic or immunologic abnormalities, among others.
> - When a patient with SLE develops neurologic symptoms, the first question that must be asked is whether the episode is a direct consequence of the inflammatory disease; an indirect effect, such as a result of an affected organ outside the nervous system or an adverse event associated with treatment; or simply an unrelated event.
> - Thrombotic events are common as a direct manifestation of SLE but may also occur as a consequence of the anticardiolipin antibody syndrome or as a secondary cardioembolic event related to involvement of the heart.
> - When neuropsychiatric manifestations are thought to be on an immunologic or inflammatory basis, the use of corticosteroids alone or in combination with immunosuppressive agents such as azathioprine or cyclophosphamide is generally recommended.

Further Reading

Bertsias GK, Boumpas DT. Pathogenesis, diagnosis and management of neuropsychiatric SLE manifestations. *Nat Rev Rheumatol* 2010; 6(6):358-367.

Brey RL. Neurologic manifestations of systemic lupus erythematosus and antiphospholipid antibody syndrome. *Continuum Lifelong Learning Neurol* 2008; 14(1):94-119.

Bruns A, Meyer O. Neuropsychiatric manifestations of systemic lupus erythematosus. *Joint Bone Spine* 2006; 73(6):639-645.

Muscal E, Brey RL. Neurologic manifestations of systemic lupus erythematosus in children and adults. *Neurol Clin* 2010; 28(1):61-73.

18 Hashimoto's Encephalopathy

A 55-year-old courthouse stenographer with a past
medical history of depression and mild hypertension
presents to her primary care physician with a 3-week
history of gradual confusion, behavioral change, and
slurred speech. Her husband reports she appears very
fatigued and "in a fog." Medications include citalopram
5 mg and hydrochlorothiazide 25 mg daily without any
recent changes. She drinks a few glasses of red wine
weekly and denies any history of tobacco or illicit drug
use. There is no history of fevers, chills, or recent
infections. On general examination, she is afebrile with a
blood pressure of 132/68 and regular pulse of 72. She is
awake and alert, but inattentive and easily distractible.
Speech is slow and mildly dysarthric but fluent. She is able
to follow simple commands, albeit with some right/left
confusion. She registers three out of three items but can
recall only two of three at one minute despite prompting.
Cranial nerve examination is normal and motor
examination demonstrates normal tone, full power, and
symmetrically normoactive reflexes except for depressed
ankle jerks. Plantar responses are mute bilaterally.

Sensory and coordination testing are grossly intact but limited because of poor cooperation. Gait is steady and symmetric. General examination is significant for mild thyromegaly. There is no evidence of meningismus. Her primary care physician refers her to the emergency room for evaluation for a subacute encephalopathy. A CT of the head is performed and demonstrates mild white matter changes consistent with small vessel occlusive disease without any acute findings. Laboratory studies demonstrate a normal complete blood count, chemistries, and urinalysis. She is seen by the neurology service and admitted for further diagnostic evaluation. Additional laboratory testing, including vitamin B12, folate, methylmalonic acid, RPR, erythrocyte sedimentation rate, and basic thyroid function tests, are normal. MRI of the brain demonstrates bilateral nonspecific subcortical T2 hyperintense white matter lesions without enhancement, and an electroencephalogram (EEG) demonstrates diffuse slowing with occasional intermittent sharp waves in the temporal regions. A lumbar puncture is performed, which reveals a lymphocytic pleocytosis of 12 cells, 88% lymphocytes, and an elevated protein of 85. Cultures and viral PCRs are negative, neuronal specific enolase and protein 14-3-3 for prion disease are negative, and cytology is benign. An anti-thyroperoxidase (TPO) antibody titer is positive.

What do you do now?

This patient presents with a subacute encephalopathy. Neurologic examination suggests involvement of several levels of the nervous system, ranging from cortical and subcortical to peripheral nerves, suggesting a widespread, systemic etiology. The differential diagnosis for a subacute encephalopathy is lengthy and includes consideration of infectious, vascular, toxic-metabolic, neurodegenerative, inflammatory, and autoimmune processes. A diagnostic workup including MR imaging, EEG, and lumbar puncture for CSF studies should be considered, in addition to laboratory testing for basic metabolic derangements such as electrolyte and liver disarray, thyroid function tests, vitamin B12 levels, and infectious processes. A primary CNS vasculitis or burgeoning subacute dementia such as early Alzheimer's, Creutzfeld-Jakob disease, and paraneoplastic syndromes also need to be considered.

In this patient, CSF studies suggest an aseptic inflammatory process and EEG suggests cortical irritability. There is systemic evidence of thyroid disease, specifically autoimmune thyroiditis, in the presence of mild thyromegaly and positive anti-TPO antibodies. Any neuropsychiatric condition occurring in the setting of probable or diagnosed autoimmune thyroiditis should raise strong suspicion for Hashimoto's encephalopathy, also known as encephalopathy associated with autoimmune thyroiditis or steroid-responsive encephalopathy with autoantibodies to thyroperoxidase (SREAT). Hashimoto's encephalopathy, first described in 1966 by Brain and colleagues, is rare, with only approximately 30 cases having been described in the neurology literature to date, and it is often misdiagnosed because of the considerable clinical and laboratory overlap with other possible causes of subacute encephalopathy. The average age of onset is late 40s, and most cases have occurred in women. MRI and CSF findings are often nonspecific. CSF oligoclonal bands have been reported but are nonspecific. Clinically, patients can demonstrate diffuse myoclonus suggesting an encephalopathy or epileptiform process. EEG is abnormal in approximately 90% of cases; however, most patients do not demonstrate significant clinical improvement with anticonvulsant therapy. Most patients present in a clinically euthyroid state and thyroid studies tend to be normal. Anti-TPO antibodies do not appear to be pathogenic, with no known CNS antigenicity shared with the corresponding thyroid gland. Antibody levels also appear to correlate poorly with disease activity. While the exact mechanism of disease in Hashimoto's encephalopathy remains unknown, an autoimmune disseminated encephalomyelitis or a vasculitic process has been postulated, although conventional cerebral angiography and transcranial Doppler ultrasounds are also typically normal.

Unlike encephalopathy associated with hypothyroidism, Hashimoto's encephalopathy improves with steroid treatment rather than thyroxine replacement. If the clinical suspicion is present and alternative etiologies have been excluded, an empiric trial of high-dose steroids should be considered, using prednisone at doses ranging from 50 mg to 150 mg daily, which produces dramatic clinical improvement within days to weeks of initiation in approximately 50% of cases. Steroids are tapered after weeks to months, with the majority of patients remaining in remission; however, relapse can occur with abrupt steroid withdrawal. In patients with steroid resistance, alternative therapeutic strategies can be considered, such as steroid-sparing immunosuppressants, plasma exchange, or intravenous immunoglobulins.

KEY POINTS TO REMEMBER

- Hashimoto's encephalopathy is a rare but potentially corticosteroid-responsive disorder and should be considered in cases of encephalopathy of unclear etiology.
- Differential diagnosis includes subacute encephalopathies such as toxic-metabolic derangements and subacute dementing illnesses such as Creutzfeld-Jakob disease, early Alzheimer's dementia, and paraneoplastic syndromes such as limbic encephalitides.
- Hashimoto's thyroiditis usually does not accompany Hashimoto's encephalopathy, and thyroid function is generally clinically normal.
- Treatment with corticosteroids is generally effective, but alternative steroid-sparing immunosuppressants should be considered in steroid-refractory cases.

Further Reading

Mijajlovic M, Mirkovic M, Dackovic J, et al. Clinical manifestations, diagnostic criteria and therapy of Hashimoto's encephalopathy: Report of two cases. *J Neurol Sci* 2010; 288:194-196.

Mocellin R, Walterfang M, Velakoulis D. Hashimoto's encephalopathy: epidemiology, pathogenesis and management. *CNS Drugs* 2007; 21(10):799-811.

Payer J, Petrovic T, Baqi L, et al. Hashimoto's encephalopathy and rare cases of hyperthyroidism (review and case report). *Endocrine Regulations* 2009; 43: 169-178.

19 Celiac Disease

A 35-year-old woman with a history of depression and irritable bowel syndrome (IBS) complains to her primary care physician of three months of memory problems, fatigue, and trouble with coordination in her limbs. In addition, she has been experiencing painful burning tingling in her hands and feet, which is most intense at night. She works as a travel agent and has been making mistakes with client schedules and computer transactions. The pain in her limbs is worse in the evening and is keeping her from getting a good night's sleep. She has never had good balance but reports she has been dropping things more easily and often stumbles during her morning walk with friends. Her IBS symptoms seem worse, with increased bloating, abdominal cramping, and loose stools. Her primary care physician orders some basic laboratory studies, including complete blood count, chemistries, liver function tests, thyroid, and vitamin B12 studies, which are essentially normal apart from a mild iron deficiency anemia, which has been chronic and attributed to heavy menses. She is referred for neurologic evaluation and on examination is found to have mild short-term memory impairment, subtle dysmetria with finger-to-nose testing, and hypoactive reflexes with flexor plantar responses. Her gait is wide-based, unsteady, and mildly dystaxic with moderate difficulty with performing tandem walking. Electromyographic (EMG) and nerve conduction velocity (NCV) studies are normal. An MRI of the brain is normal apart from subtle cerebellar atrophy. Additional laboratory testing for anti-gliadin and anti-transglutaminase antibodies is positive.

What do you do now?

Neurologic symptoms in a patient with gastrointestinal complaints should prompt consideration of systemic illnesses such as inflammatory bowel disease with associated B12 deficiency, malabsorption syndromes causing copper deficiency states, in addition to celiac, Behçet's, and Whipple's diseases, and more rarely mitochondrial diseases. As such, this patient's history of IBS should be interrogated to clarify if intrinsic bowel disease has been definitively excluded, for example by endoscopy. In the absence of structural gastrointestinal diseases, the aforementioned diseases seem less likely in this case; however, importantly, standard endoscopic procedures do not typically include enteroscopy and therefore are suboptimal as evaluation for celiac disease, which targets the small intestinal villi.

Celiac disease (CD), also known as gluten-sensitive enteropathy, is an immune-mediated illness attributed to intolerance to gluten, the storage protein of wheat, although several other proteins have been implicated. Classically, the small intestine has been considered the main target of injury; however, clinical symptoms are extremely varied and multisystemic, with a wide range of gastrointestinal and extra-intestinal manifestations, the latter including dermatologic, hematologic, endocrine, dental, and neurologic effects. CD can present at any age. There is a female-to-male predominance with a ratio of 3:1. The terms "celiac disease" and "gluten sensitivity" appear in the literature with considerable overlap. CD generally refers to biopsy evidence of small bowel villous atrophy with response of gastrointestinal symptoms such as bloating, diarrhea, and malabsorption to a gluten-free diet. Gluten sensitivity, on the other hand, describes patients with gastrointestinal symptoms responsive to gluten restriction as well as patients with abnormally elevated anti-gliadin antibodies. The degree of overlap of these entities remains unclear.

Various neurologic sequelae have been reported in CD with an estimated prevalence of 1% to 6%. Symptomatology ranges from cerebellar ataxia and peripheral sensory neuropathy, the two most commonly reported, to neuropsychiatric impairment, seizures, movement disorders, leukoencephalopathy, and myopathy. The pathogenesis of neurologic manifestations of CD remains elusive, with molecular mimicry, humoral, and T-cell mediation mechanisms implicated. Pathologic specimens have demonstrated loss of cerebellar Purkinje cells, T-cell lymphocytic infiltrates, and spinal cord posterior column degeneration.

The clinical significance of anti-gliadin antibodies has been controversial, with conflicting reports in the literature of correlation between serology and neurologic dysfunction. Recent immunocytochemical studies have demonstrated anti-gliadin antibody cross-reactivity with cerebellar Purkinje cells. In addition to anti-gliadin antibodies, anti-endomysial and anti-tissue transglutaminase autoantibodies have been reported to be both more sensitive and specific for CD, targeting smooth muscle connective tissue and an autoantigen contained within the endomysium identified as tissue transglutaminase, respectively.

Clinically, gluten ataxia generally presents with a slow, insidious progression of unsteady gait and imbalance. Patients can demonstrate evidence of concomitantly brisk reflexes or alternatively hyporeflexia in the setting of peripheral neuropathy, as well as mild cognitive dysfunction, abnormal eye movements, and myoclonus. Diagnostic evaluation should involve an MRI of the brain and spinal cord looking for cerebellar atrophy or posterior column abnormalities, respectively. In addition, EMG and NCV studies should be performed to evaluate for peripheral neuropathy. Peripheral neuropathy in CD is predominantly sensory and typically manifests with painful paresthesias involving the limbs and sometimes the face. Motor weakness is rare and often distal. Mononeuritis multiplex presentations have also been reported. Of note, CD has been identified in 5% of patients with neuropathic symptoms but normal electrodiagnostic studies. Suspected small-fiber neuropathies with no abnormalities evident on EMG and NCV studies should therefore be further pursued diagnostically with a skin biopsy, which typically demonstrates significantly decreased epidermal nerve fiber density.

Neurologic symptoms can be the presenting manifestation of CD. Duodenal biopsy in this clinical scenario has been reported to reveal evidence of classical enteropathy with pathognomonic flattened, atrophic villi despite minimal clinical gastrointestinal symptoms. A gluten-free diet can be considered in the setting of isolated neurologic disease, but clinical improvement in symptoms such as ataxia and peripheral neuropathy has been variable and conflicting, with limited data to suggest a consistent therapeutic response across patients.

- Approximately 50% of adult patients with celiac disease present with extra-intestinal manifestations, with neurologic involvement estimated to occur in 6% to 10% of patients.
- Cerebellar ("gluten") ataxia and peripheral sensory neuropathy are the most common neurologic manifestations of celiac disease.
- Anti-gliadin antibodies are moderately sensitive with low specificity for celiac disease, whereas anti-endomysial antibodies and anti-tissue-transglutaminase antibodies are highly sensitive, the former also highly specific.
- Neurologic symptoms have demonstrated variable therapeutic response to a gluten-free diet, with reports of development and even worsening despite adherence to gluten-free products.

Further Reading

Briani C, Zara G, Alaedini A, et al. Neurological complications of celiac disease and autoimmune mechanisms: A prospective study. *J Neuroimmunol* 2008; 195:171-175.

Green PHT, Alaedini A, Sander HW, et al. Mechanisms underlying celiac disease and its neurologic manifestations. *Cel Mol Life Sci* 2005; 62:791-799.

Hadjivassilou M, Sanders DS, Grunewald RA, et al. Gluten sensitivity: from gut to brain. *Lancet Neurol* 2010; 9:318-330.

20 Dermatomyositis

A 32-year-old woman was referred for neurologic consultation because of weakness in her arms and legs. For the past month she had noted difficulty climbing the subway stairs on her way to work. She also experienced difficulty performing her job as a hairdresser. She had also developed "redness" on the backs of her hands and on her upper chest. She otherwise felt well. She denied fever, weight loss, double vision or other blurring of vision, shortness of breath, chest pain or palpitations, abnormalities of bladder or bowel function, or joint pain. She had no prior neurologic or medical history. Her only medication was an oral contraceptive, which she had been taking for 5 years. The family history was negative for neurologic or neuromuscular disease and autoimmune disorders.

On physical examination, the patient was a well-developed, well-nourished young woman who did not appear ill. She was afebrile and had normal blood pressure and pulse. She had a purplish discoloration of her eyelids and a puffy appearance around her eyes. Her neck and anterior chest were erythematous.

Inspection of her hands revealed erythema over the knuckles and in the interphalangeal areas. Dilated capillary loops were noted in several nail beds. The remainder of the general physical examination was normal.

The neurologic examination revealed a normal mental status. The cranial nerves were normal. Muscle tone was normal and neither atrophy nor fasciculations were evident. Neck flexor strength was 4+ and neck extensors were 5-. Shoulder abductors and elbow flexors and extensors were 4+, but more distal arm strength was normal. In the lower extremities, hip flexors and extensors and knee flexors and extensors were 4+; more distal leg muscles were normal. Deep tendon reflexes were 2+ and symmetric. Plantar responses were flexor. Sensory examination was normal.

What do you do now?

The first step in approaching a patient with a neurologic or neuromuscular disorder is to establish the likely locus of pathology. This patient has weakness of all four extremities, which might suggest a spinal cord lesion. However, several features of the clinical syndrome argue against a myelopathy. First of all, no sensory abnormalities are present. Often a sensory level to pain and temperature will be present in a patient with myelopathy. In other cases of partial myelopathy, for instance in multiple sclerosis, signs of posterior column dysfunction, particularly diminished vibratory sensation, are evident. Although in chronic myelopathies the stretch reflexes are often hyperactive, they may be normal in a more acute or subacute situation. However, irrespective of the state of the deep tendon reflexes, pathologic reflexes, particularly the Babinski sign, may be expected. In addition, with spinal cord pathology, because of the involvement of corticospinal tracts, the pattern of weakness is such that the extensors are weaker than the flexors in the arms, and the converse is true in the legs. Often both proximal and distal muscles are affected. In this patient, the flexors and extensors were equally affected in both the arms and legs and proximal muscles were exclusively involved, a pattern that would be atypical for a myelopathy. What about the possibility of a peripheral neuropathy, such as Guillain-Barré syndrome or chronic inflammatory demyelinating polyneuropathy? Although the pattern of weakness and the absence of sensory signs would be consistent with these entities, the hallmark of the demyelinating polyneuropathies is areflexia, whereas this patient had 2+ reflexes.

This patient's physical examination is most consistent with a myopathy. The involvement of proximal muscles is characteristic of most acquired myopathies, and generally flexors and extensors in the limbs are comparably affected. Deep tendon reflexes are typically not altered and, of course, sensory findings are absent.

The clinical impression of myopathy can be further supported by electrodiagnostic studies, which should be regarded as an extension of the neurologic examination. The characteristic finding in an acquired myopathy is the presence of brief-duration small-amplitude compound muscle action potentials. In addition, increased insertional and spontaneous activity such as fibrillation potentials and positive sharp waves are typically present.

An acquired myopathy of subacute onset in a patient with no underlying disorder, in the absence of signs of systemic illness, and with no history of potentially myotoxic agents, is highly likely to be an inflammatory myositis. In this patient, the characteristic dermatologic changes of a heliotrope rash, typical V-shaped erythema (in this case affecting the neck and upper chest, but sometimes also involving the face), erythema over the knuckles and interphalangeal areas, and periungual dilated capillary loops indicate a diagnosis of dermatomyositis. The other inflammatory myositides, polymyositis, subacute necrotizing myopathy, and inclusion body myositis, all lack these unique skin features. Inclusion body myositis, in contrast to these other inflammatory myopathies, has a different pattern of weakness and is characterized by its predilection for the finger and wrist extensors and the knee extensors.

Because the inflammatory myopathies result in necrosis of muscle fibers, elevation of serum creatine kinase (CK), as well as other muscle enzymes, is usually present. However, in dermatomyositis the serum CK may be normal in as many as 20% to 30% of patients. The extent of CK elevation can be great, as much as 50 times normal. However, it is important to recognize that the CK level does not correlate with the extent of weakness. Other systemic markers of inflammation, such as erythrocyte sedimentation rate, are usually normal or only minimally elevated in dermatomyositis. A variety of myositis-specific antibodies (MSAs) occur in dermatomyositis, but generally these occur in only a minority of patients and don't have much clinical utility. An exception, however, is the anti-Jo 1 antibody, which occurs in as many as 20% of dermatomyositis patients and is associated with the presence of both interstitial lung disease and arthritis. The presence of anti-Jo 1 antibody also tends to portend a worse prognosis and a less satisfactory response to treatment.

Proof of the diagnosis of dermatomyositis can come from muscle biopsy. Perifascicular atrophy is the characteristic histologic feature of the disease, but is a late finding and is observed in fewer than half of patients. It is often absent in adults with dermatomyositis. In the perifascicular areas, small degenerating fibers are present, as well as both atrophic and nonatrophic fibers. Scattered necrotic fibers may be present, but in contrast to polymyositis and inclusion body myositis, inflammatory invasion of nonnecrotic fibers is minimal. The inflammatory infiltrate in dermatomyositis is characterized primarily by macrophages, B cells, and CD4+ cells in perivascular and perimysial regions. The CD4+ cells are predominantly plasmacytoid dendritic cells, rather than CD4+ T cells (Amato & Barohn, 2009).

The deposition of the C5b-9 or membrane attack complex on or around blood vessels is an early histologic feature of dermatomyositis, implying humoral mediation of this disease rather than the T-cell pathogenesis of polymyositis. This rather specific finding generally precedes other signs of inflammation or structural abnormalities in the affected muscles.

Dermatomyositis is not a disease that is confined to muscle. The skin manifestations have already been discussed, but other organ involvement may be associated and clinicians should be alert to this possibility. Cardiac involvement is important to recognize, and although overt clinical manifestations are rather infrequent, electrocardiographic abnormalities, including conduction defects and arrhythmias, are not uncommonly present. Interstitial lung disease occurs in 10% or more of adult dermatomyositis cases, causing dyspnea and nonproductive cough, which can occur either acutely or insidiously. The characteristic radiologic appearance is that of a diffuse reticulonodular pattern, particularly involving the lung bases. When severe, a characteristic "ground-glass" appearance is present. Restrictive defects and diminished diffusion capacity are demonstrated on pulmonary function tests and arterial hypoxemia may be present.

Gastrointestinal involvement may include dysphagia and delayed gastric emptying. A more serious vasculopathy, which can result in mucosal ulceration, gut perforation, and serious hemorrhage, occurs mostly in children. Vasculopathy can also affect other organs such as eyes, kidneys, and lungs, as well as skin and muscle.

The occurrence of an underlying malignancy is a well-recognized feature of adult, but not childhood, dermatomyositis, although its incidence varies widely (from 6% to 45%) in various series. The cancer may be detected prior to or after the diagnosis of dermatomyositis, though most often within 2 years of the clinical onset of myositis. The evaluation for malignancy, in addition to annual comprehensive history and physical examination, should include routine laboratory studies such as complete blood count, chemistries, urinalysis, and test for occult blood in the stool. The physical exam should include breast and pelvic examinations for women and testicular and prostate examinations for men. This evaluation should be supplemented by chest and abdomino-pelvic CT, and mammography in women, as well as colonoscopy for patients over the age of 50 or those with gastrointestinal symptoms. The risk of associated malignancy is lower in polymyositis than in dermatomyositis, although it may be somewhat higher than that of the general population.

The treatment of choice for both dermatomyositis and polymyositis is corticosteroid administration, despite the lack of prospective, randomized double-blind trials. By general consensus, steroids are effective in improving muscle strength and function. Most experts begin treatment with oral prednisone at a dose of 0.75 to 1.5 mg/kg (up to 100 mg) daily, but sometimes after an initial course of high-dose (1,000 mg) methylprednisolone administered daily for 3 to 5 days. After 2 to 4 weeks, the regimen may be switched to alternate-day dosing, although this may need to be delayed or accomplished more slowly in patients with more severe disease. High-dose prednisone is maintained until the patients regain normal strength or reach a plateau, generally a period of 4 to 6 months. After this, a very slow taper of steroids is initiated.

A variety of second-line immunosuppressive agents are also employed in the treatment of dermatomyositis and polymyositis, despite a paucity of controlled trials. Intravenous immunoglobulin has gained favor as a treatment for inflammatory myopathies. Other fairly widely used medications include methotrexate, azathioprine, mycophenolate mofetil, and, recently, rituximab.

Cyclophosphamide, chlorambucil, cyclosporine, tacrolimus, and the tumor necrosis factor α inhibitors infliximab and etanercept have been less frequently employed. These are usually used when patients have been poorly responsive to corticosteroids or relapse during steroid taper. The addition of immunosuppressive medications should also be considered in patients with comorbidities or severe weakness. Sometimes immunosuppressive medications are used in an attempt to minimize corticosteroid use, particularly in patients who are especially at risk for steroid complications, such as the elderly or individuals with diabetes mellitus. With proper therapy, the prognosis for recovery in both dermatomyositis (in the absence of malignancy or other severe comorbidity) and polymyositis is generally favorable.

- The characteristic dermatologic changes of a heliotrope rash, typical V-shaped erythema (in this case affecting the neck and upper chest, but sometimes also involving the face), erythema over the knuckles and interphalangeal areas, and periungual dilated capillary loops indicate a diagnosis of dermatomyositis.
- Although creatine kinase levels are characteristically elevated in dermatomyositis, they may be normal in 20% to 30% of patients.
- Dermatomyositis is not purely a disorder of muscle and skin, but rather may affect multiple organs.
- Glucocorticoids are the mainstay of treatment, but IVIg has gained favor. A variety of immunosuppressive drugs have also been used.

Further Reading

Amato AA, Barohn RJ. Evaluation and treatment of inflammatory myopathies. *J Neurol Neurosurg Psychiatry* 2009; 80(10):1060-1068.

Dalakas MC. Inflammatory muscle diseases: a critical review on pathogenesis and therapies. *Curr Opin Pharmacol* 2010; 10(3):346-352.

Mammen AL. Dermatomyositis and polymyositis: Clinical presentation, autoantibodies, and pathogenesis. *Ann NY Acad Sci* 2010; 1184:134-153.

A 40-year-old man, previously in good health, complained to his primary care physician (PCP) of diffuse muscle and joint pain. He also noted that he had lost 10 pounds in the past 2 months. The general physical examination and neurologic examination were normal. The PCP diagnosed the patient as suffering from fibromyalgia and prescribed pregabalin. Over the next 2 weeks the patient noticed gradually ascending numbness of the lower extremities, but he became particularly alarmed when he awakened one morning and found that he was unable to dorsiflex his left foot. The PCP referred the patient for neurologic evaluation. At the time of neurologic consultation, the patient reported that he had experienced intermittent fevers up to 38.5°C over the past 2 weeks and had felt unusually fatigued. His only medication was pregabalin. He denied use of alcohol or tobacco but admitted that he had been a cocaine user in his 20s. On examination, the patient's temperature was 38°C, BP was 150/100, pulse was 90 and regular. Mental status and cranial nerve examination were normal. Inspection of the patient's gait revealed suggestion of left foot drop, and the patient could not dorsiflex his left foot well on attempted heel walking. Manual muscle testing was normal throughout except for severe weakness of dorsiflexion of the left foot. Tests of coordination were normal. Sensory examination demonstrated reduced pinprick sensation to the knees bilaterally. Proprioception was intact bilaterally, but vibratory sensation was diminished in the toes bilaterally. Deep tendon reflexes were 2+ and symmetric throughout except that ankle jerks were absent bilaterally. Plantar responses were flexor.

What do you do now?

The presence of constitutional symptoms, including fever, fatigue, and diffuse muscle and joint pain, raises the suspicion of a systemic illness. The symptoms of numbness in the patient's legs and tripping are strongly suggestive of peripheral neuropathy. The immediate approach to this patient should be two-pronged, attempting on the one hand to establish the nature of the underlying illness and on the other hand to demonstrate the presence and type of peripheral neuropathy. In this previously healthy man, the likelihood is strong that the neuropathy will be etiologically related to the illness causing the systemic symptoms and signs.

The likely etiology of the constitutional symptoms is either an infectious or other inflammatory (immunologic) disorder, although a neoplastic process is also a possibility. Additional evidence of the inflammatory nature of the process can be sought through routine blood testing that includes complete blood count (CBC), erythrocyte sedimentation rate, and level of C-reactive protein. Whereas a markedly elevated white blood count with neutrophilia would suggest a bacterial infection, this is rather unlikely in view of the subacute course of the illness. Blood cultures, of course, should nonetheless be acquired in view of the fever. The presence of anemia would also suggest a chronic illness, including the possibility of vasculitis.

Confirmation of the presence of neuropathy, as well as its type, requires electrodiagnostic testing (EDT, including electromyography and nerve conduction testing). In this case, one might expect to find absent or diminished sensory nerve action potentials and perhaps mildly slowed nerve conduction velocities in the lower extremities, suggesting an axonal type of sensorimotor polyneuropathy. In addition, acutely one might find an unexcitable left peroneal nerve or, later, evidence of denervation in the muscles innervated by that nerve.

The combination of a peripheral neuropathy—especially the presence of both an axonal sensorimotor neuropathy and a mononeuropathy—with a systemic illness raises the strong possibility of vasculitis. While nervous system vasculitides occur with a variety of types and etiologies, this clinical picture strongly suggests the possibility of polyarteritis nodosa (PAN).

The most common neurologic manifestations of PAN are in the peripheral nervous system. Particularly frequent is mononeuropathy or mononeuritis multiplex—a condition in which there is discrete involvement of multiple individual nerves. This results in an asymmetric mono- or polyneuropathy, and the symptoms, which are likely due to nerve infarction, tend to develop abruptly. Conversely, a more symmetric distal polyneuropathy may evolve more slowly. Definitive diagnosis of the vascular nature of the neuropathy requires peripheral nerve biopsy, which will demonstrate inflammation throughout the walls of small and medium-sized arteries. Biopsy of more easily accessible involved tissue is often possible.

CNS manifestations also occur fairly commonly in PAN, with a reported incidence between 23% and 53%. Diffuse encephalopathy, often with seizures, is one major manifestation and is marked by rapid decline in level of consciousness. Alternatively, the patient may demonstrate focal or multifocal neurologic abnormalities, usually resulting from cerebral infarction in the hemispheres, brain stem, or cerebellum. Optic neuropathy and, less commonly, involvement of other cranial nerves may occur.

PAN is a systemic illness that most often involves the peripheral nervous system, skin, kidneys, and gastrointestinal tract. It most often affects middle-aged individuals, men more than women. The American College of Rheumatology has established a diagnostic scheme that is based on the presence of at least 3 out of 10 criteria (Table 21-1).

TABLE 21-1 **Criteria for the Diagnosis of Polyarteritis Nodosa**

1. Unintended weight loss ≥4 kg since onset of illness
2. Livedo reticularis
3. Testicular pain without other identified cause
4. Myalgias, weakness, or leg tenderness (excluding shoulder and hip girdle)
5. Mononeuropathy or polyneuropathy
6. Diastolic BP >90 mmHg
7. BUN >40 mg/dL or creatinine >1.5 mg/dL, not due to dehydration or obstruction
8. Hepatitis B virus infection
9. Arteriographic abnormality (aneurysms or occlusion of visceral arteries without other cause)
10. Biopsy-demonstrated granulocytes, with or without mononuclear leukocytes, in medium-sized arterial wall

Diagnosis of polyarteritis nodosa is based on the presence of at least 3 of the 10 criteria.
Adapted from www.rheumatology.org/practice/clinical/classification/polyart.asp (accessed May 10, 2011); original reference: Lightfoot RW Jr, Michel BA, Bloch DA, et al. The American College of Rheumatology 1990 criteria for the classification of polyarteritis nodosa. *Arthritis Rheum* 1990; 33:1088-1093.

The patient described in this case meets the criteria for PAN because of the presence of weight loss, diffuse myalgias, hypertension, and peripheral neuropathy. He should also be tested for the presence of hepatitis B surface antigen or antibody in the serum, as this is also commonly associated with the condition.

Treatment generally involves the use of corticosteroids and immunosuppressive agents such as cyclophosphamide or azathioprine. If this regimen is inadequate to control the disease or is not tolerated, alternative approaches include the use of plasma exchange, intravenous immunoglobulin, mycophenolate mofetil, or rituximab.

KEY POINTS TO REMEMBER

- The combination of a peripheral neuropathy—especially the presence of both an axonal sensorimotor neuropathy and a mononeuropathy—with a systemic illness raises the strong possibility of vasculitis.
- The most common neurologic manifestations of PAN are in the peripheral nervous system. Particularly frequent is mononeuropathy or mononeuritis multiplex—a condition in which there is discrete involvement of multiple individual nerves.
- PAN is a systemic illness that most often involves the peripheral nervous system, skin, kidneys, and gastrointestinal tract.
- Treatment generally involves the use of corticosteroids and immunosuppressive agents such as cyclophosphamide or azathioprine.

Further Reading

Burns TM, Schaublin GA, Dyck PJ. Vasculitic neuropathies. *Neurol Clin* 2007; 25(1):89-113.

Gorson KC. Vasculitic neuropathies: an update. *Neurologist* 2007; 13(1):12-19.

Minagar A, Fowler M, Harris MK, Jaffe SL. Neurologic presentations of systemic vasculitides. *Neurol Clin* 2010; 28(1):171-184.

Pettigrew HD, Teuber SS, Gershwin ME. Polyarteritis nodosa. *Compr Ther* 2007; 33(3): 144-149.

22 Myasthenia Gravis

A 28-year-old woman presents with a chief complaint of intermittent double vision. She has noted over the past two weeks that images appear horizontally separated. This sometimes lasts only a few minutes but at other times persists for hours. The symptom has been most noticeable after she has been working at the computer for hours at her job as a customer service representative. Her husband has also noticed that at times one of her eyelids may droop. The patient has also noted on two recent occasions at the end of long meals at a restaurant that she choked when drinking a glass of water. She has had no significant past medical history and her family history is unremarkable. Her only medication is an oral contraceptive. She has never been pregnant. She does not smoke, drinks alcohol only occasionally, and does not use illicit drugs. She has had no recent travel.

Her neurologic examination reveals a normal mental status. She has obvious ptosis of the left eye. Pupils are 4 mm in diameter, round, and reactive to light. No relative afferent papillary defect is observed and funduscopy is normal. On extraocular muscle testing, the left eye does not move fully medially and she notes double vision when she looks to the right. Vertical eye movements seem normal. No nystagmus is noted. The remainder of the cranial nerve examination is normal. Her gait is normal. She has no weakness on manual muscle testing and muscle tone is normal. Coordination and sensory testing reveals no abnormalities. The deep tendon reflexes are 2+ and symmetric throughout and plantar responses are flexor.

What do you do now?

Most important at this time is to make an accurate diagnosis. This patient's complaints and physical examination findings of left ptosis and left medial rectus palsy might suggest the possibility of a left III nerve palsy. However, the lack of pupillary involvement makes a compressive III nerve palsy unlikely. A pupil-sparing III nerve palsy, as seen, for example, in diabetes mellitus, would be unusual in a 28-year-old woman who is otherwise completely healthy. Furthermore, the absence of involvement of other muscles innervated by CN III argues against this possibility.

A diagnosis of multiple sclerosis (MS) should certainly be in the differential of a young woman presenting with double vision. The failure of adduction of her left eye, in the absence of other extraocular motility disturbances, suggests the possibility of a left internuclear ophthalmoplegia. However, usually with an internuclear ophthalmoplegia, the abducting eye manifests horizontal nystagmus, which was absent in this case. In addition, significant ptosis is unusual in MS.

Most noteworthy, the intermittency of this patient's symptoms, especially occurring at times that the affected muscles have been working for prolonged periods of time, is not characteristic of MS and raises the strong possibility of a diagnosis of myasthenia gravis (MG), a disorder that particularly affects young women and older men. In addition to the ocular symptoms and signs, the patient has had two occurrences of dysphagia, raising the likelihood that her disorder involves other muscle groups besides those involving the eyes.

What should be done to support and ultimately confirm a diagnosis of MG? First, some additional testing at the bedside might be helpful. Fatiguing maneuvers are often helpful in eliciting or exaggerating physical signs. For example, having the patient sustain upgaze for 30 to 60 seconds may enhance ptosis or elicit a medial rectus weakness. Similarly, asking the patient to sustain abduction of the arms for 120 seconds may demonstrate weakness. In a phenomenon known as "enhanced ptosis," when the ptotic eyelid is manually elevated, ptosis in the opposite eye may become manifest or worsen. In addition, in MG, local cooling of the affected lid may improve the ptosis.

A positive edrophonium test may also strongly support a diagnosis of MG. In this test, edrophonium, a short-acting acetylcholine esterase inhibitor, is administered and the examiner looks for improvement in a sentinel sign. Successful and convincing test results require the presence of a clearly discernible improvement in a sentinel clinical sign, such as ptosis or a particular obviously paretic eye muscle. Gastrointestinal side effects such as excess salivation, nausea, and abdominal cramps may occur with administration of edrophonium. More importantly, rarely hypotension and bradycardia may develop, so atropine should be available if the latter persists.

The pathophysiology of MG relates to a loss of functional acetylcholine receptors (AChR) on the postsynaptic membrane of the neuromuscular junction caused by the presence of antibodies to the AChR in this autoimmune disorder. This results in a decrease in the magnitude of the endplate potential (EPP) and a reduction in the safety factor of neuromuscular transmission. Normally, the safety factor for neuromuscular transmission is several times greater than necessary to generate a muscle action potential. As a result, repetitive nerve stimulation (at a frequency of 2 to 5 Hz) has no significant effect in normal muscle; however, in MG, because of the diminished EPP resulting from the loss of functional AChRs, repetitive nerve stimulation results in a decremental response of the compound muscle action potential. Thus, demonstration of a decremental response of greater than 10% to repetitive nerve stimulation is strong evidence for the diagnosis of MG. Although the sensitivity of repetitive nerve stimulation is reasonably high (53% to 100%) in generalized MG, it is quite low in pure ocular myasthenia (10% to 17%). Another specialized test, known as single-fiber EMG, is highly sensitive for the diagnosis of MG, but it is less readily available.

The presence in the serum of antibodies reactive with the AChR is considered specific for acquired MG. Most widely detected are AChR-binding antibodies, which are found in 80% to 85% of patients with generalized MG but in only about half of the patients with purely ocular MG. A subpopulation of patients with MG who are negative for anti-AChR antibodies demonstrate the presence of anti-muscle specific receptor tyrosine kinase (MuSK) antibodies (about 40%). MuSK antibodies are rarely present in patients with ocular MG. Patients with MG associated with MuSK antibodies tend to have an atypical presentation in which facial, bulbar, neck, and respiratory muscles are often significantly involved, whereas ocular muscles are often spared.

The thymus gland presumably plays an important role in the development of MG, yet the specifics are poorly understood. More than half the MG patients who are AChR-antibody positive have thymic hyperplasia, and, of particular importance, 10% to 15% will harbor a thymoma, generally benign but occasionally malignant. Because of this, patients with MG should undergo chest CT scanning. The issue of thymectomy will be discussed below.

The treatment of MG encompasses both symptomatic treatment and immunologic therapies aimed at altering the natural history of the disease. Symptomatic therapy essentially consists of the use of cholinesterase inhibitors, mainly pyridostigmine. Dosing optimization must be individualized, but the usual starting dose in adults is 30 to 60 mg every 4 hours. Administration of more than 120 mg every 4 hours is seldom effective and may actually worsen weakness. Muscarinic side effects of cholinesterase inhibitors may be troublesome. These include gastrointestinal manifestations such as abdominal cramping, diarrhea, nausea and vomiting, as well as excessive sweating and bronchial or nasal secretions. The presence of such adverse effects is generally an indication for dosage reduction.

The mainstay of treatment to alter the disease course of myasthenia gravis is immunologically directed therapy. This can be considered as short-term or acute strategies to induce remission or long-term strategies to decrease the likelihood of disease exacerbation. Plasma exchange (PLEX), also known as plasmapheresis, is often employed in patients who have experienced sudden worsening of their disease, sometimes to the point of myasthenic crisis. It is also used prior to surgery, particularly thymectomy (see below), with the aim of decreasing perioperative morbidity and of optimizing the patient's condition prior to the surgery. Sometimes plasmapheresis is administered in combination with high-dose corticosteroids to try to mitigate the worsening that sometimes occurs with that therapy.

Intravenous immunoglobulin (IVIg) is often used in similar situations to those for which PLEX is employed. Recent studies have suggested that IVIg is most effective and should probably be reserved for patients with moderate to severe myasthenic symptoms, especially when a rapid treatment response is urgent. Treatment is initiated at a total dose of 2 g/kg, administered over 2 to 5 days. This is followed by maintenance therapy, typically at a dose of 0.5 to 1.0 g/kg, often administered monthly.

Corticosteroids remain the most widely used immune-mediated therapy in MG. Although definitive randomized controlled trials have not been reported, prednisone is generally regarded as effective in inducing significant improvement in a high percentage of patients. In a large observational study, Pascuzzi et al. (1984) reported that prednisone induced complete remission in 28%, marked improvement with normal activities of daily living in 53%, moderate improvement in 15%, and no improvement in only 5%. Prednisone is often initiated at a relatively high dose of 1.0 to 1.5 mg/kg, which is maintained for several months, followed by a very slow taper with close clinical observation. Many patients need to remain on at least a low dose of steroids for many years. It is important for clinicians to be aware that the initiation of high-dose corticosteroid therapy is frequently accompanied by clinical worsening before the patient begins to improve. Thus, such treatment needs to be accomplished in a hospital, sometimes in an intensive care setting, as patients (8.6% in the Pascuzzi series) may require intubation over the first 5 to 7 days. Alternatively, some experts prefer to administer PLEX or IVIg with the steroids, as noted above.

Because of the well-known and potentially serious consequences of long-term corticosteroid administration, a number of other immunosuppressive medications have been employed in the treatment of MG as "steroid-sparing" agents. They have also been used when steroid therapy has been insufficiently effective. Perhaps the most widely used drugs for this purpose have been azathioprine and, more recently, mycophenolate mofetil. Although controlled trials have not been reported, both agents appear to induce improvement in a high percentage of patients. The response to both drugs may be delayed, but perhaps less so with mycophenolate mofetil, as the lag with azathioprine may be as long as a year. Details of the use of the wide variety of immunosuppressants for the treatment of MG is beyond the scope of this discussion, but the other agents that are employed include cyclophosphamide, cyclosporine, tacrolimus, and rituximab.

Based on the presumed role of the thymus in the pathophysiology of MG, thymectomy had been performed as a therapeutic measure for nearly 70 years. Despite this long history, the benefits of the therapy have not been clearly established. This may be in part because an effect may not become evident until a very long time after surgery. Currently an international prospective, single-blind, randomized trial is ongoing in an attempt to establish whether the procedure is effective.

KEY POINTS TO REMEMBER

- Fatigability and variability of muscle strength are the hallmarks of MG, which often tends to particularly affect ocular and bulbar muscles.
- Decremental response of greater than 10% on repetitive nerve stimulation is the characteristic finding on electrodiagnostic testing.
- The treatment of MG encompasses both symptomatic treatment and immunologic therapies aimed at altering the natural history of the disease. Symptomatic therapy essentially consists of the use of cholinesterase inhibitors, mainly pyridostigmine.
- Corticosteroids remain the most widely used immune-mediated therapy in MG. It is important for clinicians to be aware that the initiation of high-dose corticosteroid therapy is frequently accompanied by clinical worsening before the patient begins to improve.

Further Reading

Farrugia ME, Vincent A. Autoimmune mediated neuromuscular junction defects. *Curr Opin Neurol* 2010; 23(5):489-495.

Guptill JT, Sanders DB. Update on muscle-specific tyrosine kinase antibody positive myasthenia gravis. *Curr Opin Neurol* 2010; 23(5):530-535.

Meriggioli MN. Myasthenia gravis: Immunopathogenesis, diagnosis, and management. *Continuum Lifelong Learning Neurol* 2009; 15(1):35-62.

Pascuzzi RM, Coslett HB, Johns TR. Long-term corticosteroid treatment of myasthenia gravis: report of 116 patients. *Ann Neurol* 1984; 15(3):291-298.

Sanders DB, Evoli A. Immunosuppressive therapies in myasthenia gravis. *Autoimmunity* 2010; 43(5-6):428-435.

23 Lambert-Eaton Myasthenia Syndrome

A 54-year-old man with hypercholesterolemia and a 25-pack/year history of tobacco use presented to his primary care physician (PCP) with 6 months of progressive weakness involving his lower extremities in addition to occasional diplopia. He reports significant difficulty rising from a chair and ascending stairs, although he reports his legs feel stronger as he reaches the top of the staircase. He also complains of occasional urinary hesitancy and nonvertiginous lightheadedness with abrupt changes in posture. He denies any recent weight loss, night sweats, dyspnea, or cough. His only medication is atorvastatin. Complete blood counts, chemistries, liver function testing, and thyroid and vitamin B12 levels were normal. CPK and anti-Jo levels and erythrocyte sedimentation rate are normal. Despite discontinuation of his statin, there was no improvement in his symptoms; therefore, his PCP referred him for evaluation. On neurologic examination, he had full extraocular movements, without pupillary asymmetry or ptosis, and an otherwise normal cranial nerve examination. Motor examination revealed normal bulk with moderate proximal muscle weakness primarily involving his hip flexors bilaterally, normoactive deep tendon reflexes, flexor plantar responses, and a slow but steady narrow-based gait. No fasciculations were observed on inspection, and sensory testing was intact to all modalities. General examination revealed a thin but well-nourished man. A plain chest radiograph performed 6 months prior demonstrated bilaterally hyperinflated lungs with flattened diaphragm and no evidence of any mediastinal masses. An edrophonium test was performed in the neurologist's office, and the results were indeterminate. An electromyographic/nerve conduction velocity (EMG/NCV) study demonstrated post-exercise facilitation without evidence of polyneuropathy or myopathy, suggesting a presynaptic neuromuscular junction defect.

What do you do now?

The initial differential diagnosis for this patient's complaint of progressive proximal lower extremity weakness is extensive. The neurologic examination, however, does not demonstrate evidence of myelopathy, radiculopathy or polyneuropathy, thereby increasing the suspicion for either a myopathic or neuromuscular junction (NMJ) disorder. A statin-induced myopathy was considered, but CPK levels were normal and there was no improvement with discontinuation of atorvastatin. A rheumatologic process such as polymyalgia rheumatica could be considered, but there were no significant complaints of pain and the erythrocyte sedimentation rate was normal. In addition, toxic-metabolic–related myopathies such as those caused by thyroid dysfunction or electrolyte disturbances were excluded.

The additional bulbar complaint of episodic diplopia raises suspicion for disorders of the neuromuscular junction, such as myasthenia gravis (MG) or Lambert-Eaton myasthenia syndrome (LEMS). Clinically, findings of MG and LEMS can be difficult to differentiate. MG tends to affect predominantly extraocular muscles and bulbar function, with infrequent extremity weakness. Conversely, LEMS patients rarely present with bulbar weakness and more often demonstrate insidious proximal limb weakness, primarily affecting the lower extremities. Weakness in MG is generally fatigable with repetitive exercise, whereas LEMS patients conversely experience an augmentation in strength within the initial seconds of maximum exercise effort. Electrophysiological studies can be critical in helping to differentiate between MG and LEMS when clinical findings are indistinct and overlapping, as in this patient presenting with both extraocular and limb weakness. However, the post-exercise augmentation in strength is suspicious for LEMS.

LEMS, an autoimmune-mediated disorder of the NMJ, was first described in 1951 as severe muscle weakness in a patient with bronchial neoplasm, which resolved after tumor removal. In 1956, Lambert described the electromyographic features of LEMS, distinguishing it from MG. LEMS is associated with autoantibodies to P/Q-type voltage-gated calcium channels (VGCC) present on the presynaptic membrane of the NMJ, which can be either paraneoplastic or non-paraneoplastic. These antibodies have also been implicated in cerebellar ataxia, occasionally observed in LEMS patients. In paraneoplastic LEMS, VGCC antibodies are associated with small cell lung cancer (SCLC) in 50% to 60% of cases. In a large prospective study, 3% of patients with SCLC were found to have paraneo-plastic LEMS. Patients with SCLC have been reported to demonstrate a more rapidly progressive LEMS, in contrast to patients without tumors. Interestingly, however, patients with antibody-positive LEMS appear to have a better survival rate, suggesting a protective role for these antibodies, although studies involving larger numbers of patients are necessary to confirm this observation. A second subset of autoantibodies to SOX proteins, a group of developmental transcription factors with an integral role in neurogenesis, have been shown to further discriminate between LEMS associated with SCLC and non-paraneoplastic LEMS, although no correlation with prognosis has been made in this setting. Lymphoproliferative disorders are also occasionally found to be the cause of paraneoplastic LEMS. Non-paraneoplastic LEMS has a greater incidence of associated autoimmune disorders, such as vitiligo and thyroid conditions.

The most common initial symptom of LEMS is difficulty ambulating secondary to proximal leg weakness. Proximal upper extremity weakness is also a frequent complaint; however, ptosis and occasional diplopia are more often seen with MG. In rare instances, dyspnea is reported secondary to involvement of respiratory musculature in LEMS. Neurologic examination typically reveals augmentation of strength during the initial period of maximum effort as well as hypoactive reflexes and post-tetanic potentiation. Dysautonomias are also very common, including constipation, erectile dysfunction, and dry mouth. Electromyography reveals an abnormally small compound muscle action potential whose amplitude increases or facilitates following maximum voluntary contraction or with high-frequency electrical stimulation. This neurophysiologic phenomenon occurs secondary to the reduced quantal release of the neurotransmitter acetylcholine at the presynaptic membrane. Patients sometimes respond to intravenous edrophonium, but generally not as clearly as MG patients.

The management of LEMS involves investigation for an occult tumor. If CT scanning of the thorax is unremarkable, a whole-body PET scan should be strongly considered, as tumor removal is associated with significant clinical improvement, attributed to removal of the source of antigenic-driven antibody response. In addition, the symptomatic therapy of choice is 3,4-diaminoyridine (3,4-DAP), which acts by blocking the presynaptic voltage-gated potassium channels to prolong the action potential and increase calcium ion influx to the nerve terminal. Two randomized controlled studies have demonstrated both subjective and neurophysiologic benefit from this 3,4-DAP, which, apart from mild perioral and limb paresthesias, is generally very well tolerated. Occasional symptomatic improvement has also been described with pyridostigmine, but not as impressively as seen in MG patients. In patients who remain symptomatic despite tumor removal and 3,4-DAP, trials of corticosteroids, steroid-sparing immunosuppressants such as azathioprine and cyclosporine, as well as courses of intravenous immunoglobulin or plasma exchange, can be considered, although only short-term benefits appear to be conferred by the two latter approaches, without evidence supporting their role as long-term maintenance therapies.

KEY POINTS TO REMEMBER

- LEMS is an autoimmune-mediated disorder of the NMJ, which involves autoantibodies to P/Q-type voltage-gated calcium channels on the presynaptic membrane.
- The characteristic clinical features of LEMS include proximal muscle weakness, dysautonomias, and augmentation of muscle strength during initial voluntary activation.
- The majority (60%) of LEMS cases are paraneoplastic and associated with small cell lung cancers, with good response to tumor removal.
- In cases with severe weakness or refractory to tumor removal, immunotherapies such as corticosteroids, immunosuppressants, intravenous immunoglobulin, and plasma exchange can be considered.

Further Reading

Farrugia ME, Vincent A. Autoimmune mediated neuromuscular junction defects. *Curr Opin Neurol* 2010; 23:489-495.

Newson-Davis J. Lambert-Eaton myasthenic syndrome. *Rev Neurol (Paris)* 2004; 160:177-180.

Quartel A, Turbeville S, Lounsbury. Current therapy for Lambert-Eaton myasthenic syndrome: development of 3,4-diaminopyridine phosphate salt as first-line symptomatic treatment. *Curr Med Res Opin* 2010; 26:1363-1375.

24 Acute Inflammatory Demyelinating Polyneuropathy (Guillain-Barré Syndrome)

A 60-year-old man presents to the emergency department because of weakness of his legs. He was in his usual state of health until 3 days before, when he began to notice some aching pain in his middle and lower back. A day later he began to experience some tingling sensations in his feet and lower legs and the next day he had some difficulty climbing stairs, but he ascribed this to fatigue from an arduous workout he had done earlier. The following morning, however, he noticed definite weakness in his legs and found that he needed to push off with his hands in order to arise from the toilet seat. He had experienced no difficulty with urinary or bowel function. He was a business executive who was in good health except for hypercholesterolemia, for which he took atorvastatin, his only medication. He had experienced no recent febrile illness. He denied recent travel, but he had been on a camping and fishing trip the previous weekend with his son and grandsons. He does not smoke and drinks two glasses of wine once or twice a week.

Physical examination demonstrated a well-developed, well-nourished man in no acute distress. Blood pressure was 115/75, pulse 72 and regular, and respiratory rate was 12. On neurologic examination the patient had a normal mental status. Cranial nerve examination was normal. Muscle strength was normal in the upper extremities. Lower extremity power was 4/5 in both iliopsoas and both quadriceps muscles. The hamstrings were 4+/5 bilaterally and ankle dorsiflexors were 5−/5. Muscle tone was normal. No atrophy or fasciculations were evident. He was able to walk independently, but slowly and with a waddling quality. Finger-to-nose testing, rapid alternating movements in the upper extremities, and heel-knee-shin tests were normal. Sensory examination revealed intact pinprick sensation and joint position sense. He perceived vibration for only 5 seconds in the big toes bilaterally. Deep tendon reflexes were 2+ in the upper extremities, trace ankle jerks, and absent knee jerks. Plantar responses were flexor bilaterally.

What do you do now?

This patient's clinical picture is most suggestive of an acute polyneuropathy. The presence of back pain and paraparesis should raise concern about the possibility of myelopathy from spinal cord compression. However, the severely reduced to absent deep tendon reflexes in the legs, the lack of Babinski sign, the absence of a sensory level to pinprick, and the normal bladder and bowel function make this diagnosis unlikely. The presence of muscle weakness in a patient taking atorvastatin raises the possibility of a statin-induced myopathy. That condition would not have been associated with sensory complaints, reduction of vibratory sensation, and loss of deep tendon reflexes. The presence of muscle weakness in a person who has recently been in the woods should prompt a search for a tick because of the possibility of tick paralysis, but usually circumstances suggest the possibility of exposure to the arthropod.

Similarly, envenomation from a black widow spider bite can cause muscle paralysis. The spiders tend to lurk in dark, damp environments such as campground outhouses, where they might bite a man in the genital area. The patient denied any bites, and spider venom should not cause sensory changes. It typically does cause muscle and chest tightness and often abdominal pain, cramping, or nausea.

Another cause of acute muscle weakness resembling acute inflammatory polyneuropathy is the mosquito-borne West Nile virus. The neurologic complications of West Nile virus infection of anterior horn cells in spinal cord and in brain neurons as well characteristically results in asymmetric disease (as was characteristic for polio years ago), thus helping to distinguish it from the more typically symmetric acute polyneuropathy of GBS. Serologic evidence for this infection should be sought. The possibility of acute neuroborreliosis (Lyme disease) should also be investigated by antibody testing, but this etiology is unlikely in the absence of cutaneous or rheumatologic symptoms.

This patient actually presents with a classical picture of acute inflammatory demyelinating polyneuropathy (AIDP), also known as Guillain-Barré syndrome (GBS). The disease often begins with a prodrome of back or extremity pain, and this is followed by the development of mild sensory symptoms, which usually does not prompt the patient to seek medical attention. The development of motor weakness, which most often begins in the lower extremities, frequently ascends, and characteristically involves proximal muscles, usually compels the patient to seek medical care. A hallmark of the disorder is the loss of deep tendon reflexes in weak muscles. It is important to recognize, however, that deep tendon reflexes may be preserved in muscles that have normal strength or minimal weakness. Despite the common sensory symptoms, the sensory examination is often normal or shows mild impairment of proprioception or vibratory sensation, as in this patient.

In as many as 70% of patients, an antecedent viral or bacterial infection has occurred that is suspected to have triggered the neurologic syndrome. Generally, GBS occurs 1 to 4 weeks after the infectious illness, which has usually resolved before the onset of neurologic symptoms. In most cases, the infectious agent for the preceding illness is not identified. Cytomegalovirus and Epstein-Barr viral infections are among the most commonly recognized viral illnesses preceding the development of GBS. In addition, human immunodeficiency virus is associated with GBS, especially at the time of seroconversion. The most frequently occurring bacterial pathogen associated with the development of GBS, although mainly of the axonal variant of the syndrome, is *Campylobacter jejuni*, a common cause of gastroenteritis throughout the world. However, in the United States, the actual risk of developing GBS after *C. jejuni* infection has been estimated to be only about 0.1%.

The pathology of classical GBS, as reflected by its alternative term AIDP, is characterized by lymphocytic infiltrates in peripheral nerves and spinal roots, with subsequent stripping of myelin by macrophages. The speculative hypothesis of *molecular mimickry* suggests that an antecedent infectious agent shares antigenic homology with components of the peripheral nerves.

A highly characteristic feature of GBS is the presence of so-called cytoalbuminologic dissociation, which refers to the finding in the CSF of a low cell count (mononuclear cells) in the presence of an elevated protein level. Therefore, this patient should undergo lumbar puncture, although sometimes this typical CSF pattern is absent very early in the course of the illness.

Electrodiagnostic studies should be performed very early in patients with suspected GBS because they provide critical information for both diagnosis and prognosis. Because the pathology of AIDP, as indicated by this term, is primarily demyelinating, nerve conduction studies typically show slowing of conduction and partial or complete conduction block in motor nerves. Similar findings are often present in median and ulnar nerves, though sparing of the sural nerve is often seen. The ultimate prognosis of GBS often depends on the extent of axonal damage, which can be suggested on electrodiagnostic testing by the finding of significant reduction of compound muscle action potentials.

Patients with GBS need close observation in the hospital. While a spectrum of severity of the disorder exists, patients with rapidly progressing weakness or any sign of respiratory involvement should be managed in an intensive care unit (ICU). Indeed, it was the development of the modern ICU that has been most instrumental in reducing the mortality rate to its current level of under 5%.

Close monitoring of the patient for signs of respiratory compromise is imperative. This can generally be done with bedside spirometry, as well as pulse oximetry. Intubation should be done electively rather than waiting for a crisis. The patient should be intubated when the vital capacity (VC) decreases to about 1,000 mL, or even earlier, if the VC is declining rapidly or if significant oropharyngeal weakness that may interfere with the handling of secretions is present.

Another important issue for the management of patients with GBS is the fact that their autonomic nervous system is often compromised. Thus, they are subject to wide swings in blood pressure, either hypertension or hypotension, as well as cardiac arrhythmias. Great care should be taken in maneuvering patients to avoid sudden positional shifts that may precipitate dramatic changes in BP and to adequately oxygenate patients before suctioning, while monitoring them closely. Bladder and bowel dysfunction also commonly occurs with severe GBS. Adynamic ileus develops in about half of patients, and clinicians must be vigilant in recognizing and managing this condition, which will require suspension of gut feeding.

Lying in a hospital bed, especially in an ICU, motionless and unable to communicate verbally if intubated, is a terrifying experience for patients. Staff and visitors need to remember that the patient, though paralyzed, is usually fully conscious, mentally intact, and aware of everything that is said around him or her. Diligent efforts must be made to enable means of communication with the patient, for example through systems of sign boards and eye blinks. Anxiolytic medications may be helpful in some cases.

Although GBS is generally a self-limited disease, a major therapeutic breakthrough occurred more than three decades ago with the demonstration that plasma exchange is effective in accelerating recovery. Plasma exchange is usually conducted by exchanging one plasma volume of 50 mL/kg in each of five treatments over the course of 2 weeks. The treatment is best initiated within 2 weeks of the onset of symptoms but should not be started more than 4 weeks after onset. After initially improving, approximately 10% of patients treated with plasma exchange will worsen within 2 weeks. These patients should receive additional exchanges or, alternatively, intravenous immunoglobulin (IVIg), as described below.

Following the demonstration of the utility of plasma exchange, studies found that administration of IVIg was as effective as plasma exchange in hastening improvement in nonambulatory patients who received treatment within 2 weeks of onset of symptoms. The usual dose is 2g/kg divided over 2 to 5 days. Because IVIg is more readily administered than plasma exchange, most practitioners prefer it as initial therapy. Contraindications include low serum IgA levels, advanced renal disease, hypertension, or hyperosmolar state. As with plasma exchange, worsening may occur following initial improvement in a small proportion of patients. This situation usually improves with repeat IVIg administration. No advantage is gained by the sequential administration of plasma exchange followed by IVIg. Furthermore, the use of corticosteroids as sole therapy for GBS has been shown to be ineffective.

In general, the long-term prognosis of patients with GBS is good. However, approximately 20% have a protracted recovery phase and are left with significant functional disability.

KEY POINTS TO REMEMBER

- The disease often begins with a prodrome of back or extremity pain, and this is followed by the development of mild sensory symptoms, which usually does not prompt the patient to seek medical attention. This is followed by more dramatic muscle weakness that compels the patient to seek medical attention.

- A hallmark of the disorder is the loss of deep tendon reflexes in weak muscles. It is important to recognize, however, that deep tendon reflexes may be preserved in muscles that have normal strength or minimal weakness.

- A highly characteristic feature of GBS is the presence of so-called cyto-albuminologic dissociation, which refers to the finding in the CSF of a low cell count (mononuclear cells) in the presence of an elevated protein level.

- Plasmapheresis and administration of IVIg are the treatments of choice for GBS. Although they are equally effective, the latter is preferred because it is easier to use.

Further Reading

Hughes RA, Swan AV, van Doorn PA. Corticosteroids for Guillain-Barré syndrome. *Cochrane Database Syst Rev* 2010;17(2):CD001446.

Linker RA, Gold R. Use of intravenous immunoglobulin and plasma exchange in neurological disease. *Curr Opin Neurol* 2008; 2(13):358-365.

Van Doorn PA, Ruts L, Jacobs BC. Clinical features, pathogenesis, and treatment of Guillain-Barrȅ syndrome. *Lancet Neurol* 2008; 7(10):939-950.

Vucic S, Kiernan MC, Cornblath DR. Guillain-Barrȅ syndrome: an update. *J Clin Neurosci* 2009;16(6): 733-741.

Chronic Inflammatory
Demyelinating
Polyneuropathy

A 58-year-old man presented for evaluation of numbness
and weakness in his legs. He had noticed gradually
worsening weakness for about 6 months, but attributed
this to the fact that he had stopped working out because
he was very busy at work and felt too fatigued to
exercise. He seeks consultation, however, because he has
recently had an upper respiratory infection with low-
grade fever, which was associated with a substantial
worsening of his strength. He also had begun to notice
some numbness of his feet. He reported no difficulties
with his arms, no visual disturbances, no facial numbness
or weakness, and no dysphagia. He had some mild aching
in his calves, but no other pain. He had no problems with
bladder or bowel function. He had never previously had
any neurologic problems.

The patient's past medical history was unremarkable.
His only medication was atorvastatin 10 mg daily. He had
never smoked, drinks a glass or two of wine
approximately once a week, and has never used any illicit
drugs. He works as an accountant. The patient was
adopted and he does not know anything about his

biological family. He has a daughter age 35 and a son age 32, both healthy.

General physical examination revealed normal vital signs and no other abnormalities. On neurologic examination, the mental status and cranial nerves were normal. His gait had a waddling quality and he had difficulty arising from a chair. Muscle inspection did not reveal wasting or fasciculations. Muscle tone was normal. On manual muscle testing, strength was normal in the arms. In the legs, hip flexors and extensors as well as knee flexors and extensors were 4/5. Ankle dorsiflexion was 4+ and plantarflexion was minimally weak. Finger-nose-finger testing, rapid alternating movements, and heel-knee-shin tests were all normal. No tremor was present. Romberg test was negative. Sensory examination demonstrated mild impairment of proprioception and moderate impairment of vibratory sensation in the toes. Deep tendon reflexes were 1+ in the upper extremities and absent in the lower extremities. Plantar responses were flexor.

What do you do now?

As with any neurologic problem, the initial task is to establish the anatomic localization of the problem. Bilateral lower extremity weakness almost always implies pathology in the spinal cord or in peripheral nerve–neuromuscular junction–muscle complex. The leg areflexia and absence of Babinski sign, the lack of a sensory level to pain and temperature, and the normal bladder and bowel function all argue strongly against structural pathology in the spinal cord. The absence of atrophy and fasciculation makes a disease of the anterior horn cells, such as amyotrophic lateral sclerosis, highly unlikely.

The finding of areflexia in the lower extremities is very important in this case, as it makes the clinical scenario much more likely to be due to peripheral nerve disease than to muscle or neuromuscular junction disease. In addition, the complaint of numbness of the feet is significant and the findings on the sensory examination favor the diagnosis of peripheral neuropathy, despite the absence of objective sensory signs on the neurologic examination. Neither neuromuscular junction disorders, such as myasthenia gravis, nor primary muscle disease would be accompanied by involvement of sensory pathways.

Having established the presumptive locus of pathology as the peripheral nerves, one should then consider what type of peripheral neuropathy is present. The subacute onset in a patient in the sixth decade of life makes the possibility of a hereditary neuropathy extremely unlikely. Many of the typical axonal polyneuropathies, such as those associated with diabetes mellitus or alcoholism, affect the longest axons first and therefore cause initial symptoms in the distal lower extremities. In addition, they are typically characterized earlier and more prominently by sensory symptoms and signs than by significant motor weakness. In contrast, acquired demyelinating inflammatory polyneuropathies more frequently involve proximal muscles, have more prominent motor than sensory symptoms and signs, and most often involve lower extremities more than upper ones, although an ascending pattern of weakness is often seen. Thus, this patient's illness is likely in this category, which includes both acute and chronic forms. The former, which is discussed in Chapter 24, reaches its nadir in not more than 4 weeks and usually in less than that. Chronic forms, on the other hand, tend to progress over many months and may take either a steadily progressive or relapsing course. Relapses or significant worsening, as in this case, are often precipitated by even minor infections. Because this patient's symptoms include both motor (predominant) and sensory features, he is likely experiencing chronic inflammatory demyelinating (sensorimotor) polyneuropathy (CIDP). Occasionally, the acquired chronic inflammatory neuropathies may be selectively motor or sensory.

Confirmation of the likelihood of demyelinating polyneuropathy can be obtained by electrodiagnostic study, which should include all four limbs. Marked slowing of conduction velocity is found in the vast majority of cases. Because the inflammatory demyelinating process is patchy, the characteristic electrophysiologic feature is non-uniform slowing of motor conduction and accompanying partial conduction block. Significant diminution of the amplitude of compound muscle action potentials also usually occurs because of the combination of temporal dispersion and the secondary loss of axons that generally happens in the chronic disease. Because of this axonal involvement, electromyography will typically show signs of denervation and partial reinnervation, such as fibrillation potentials and giant, long-duration, polyphasic potentials.

The CSF examination is an important part of the diagnostic evaluation in a patient suspected to have CIDP. As in acute inflammatory demyelinating polyneuropathy (Guillain-Barré syndrome), the typical finding is cytoalbuminologic dissociation—that is, few cells (usually <10 mononuclear cells) are present in combination with an elevated protein level (>60 mg/dL). The presence of more than 50 cells should raise the possibility of an underlying disorder such as human immunodeficiency virus infection or a hematologic malignancy. Occasionally CIDP is associated with a plasma cell dyscrasia or a monoclonal gammopathy, so workup, including immunoelectrophoresis, should be conducted to exclude these entities.

Usually the investigations described above are sufficient to make the diagnosis of CIDP. Occasionally, however, biopsy is necessary to confirm the condition by demonstrating the characteristic pattern of segmental demyelination and recurrent remyelination with the presence of infiltrating macrophages.

Once the diagnosis is established, long-term therapy for this chronic, and frequently relapsing, disease must be instituted. For years, corticosteroids were the mainstay of therapy, usually requiring fairly high doses (e.g. often initiated at a dose of 60 or more mg/day) for a prolonged period.

Some experts have preferred to begin with high-dose intravenous methyl-prednisolone (e.g., 1,000 mg for 3 to 5 days, followed by weekly infusions of a similar dose) before switching patients to oral corticosteroids and eventually, after remission is achieved, beginning a slow taper. In recent years, however, many experts have preferred to use intravenous immunoglobulin (IVIg) either alone or in combination with corticosteroids as first-line therapy. A randomized double-blind placebo-controlled trial of IVIg, beginning with a loading dose of 2 g/kg administered over 2 to 4 days and followed with a maintenance dose of 1 g/kg over 1 to 2 weeks given every 3 weeks for up to 24 weeks, showed a statistically significant benefit of IVIg. At the conclusion of the 24-week trial, 54% of the IVIG group showed improvement in disability scores, compared to 21% of the placebo group. In addition, the former group showed only a 13% relapse rate compared to a 45% rate in the latter during a 24-week extension study. This trial led to the approval of the use of IVIg for CIDP by the U.S. Food and Drug Administration in 2008. For pure motor CIDP, IVIg is now regarded as the preferred initial choice. Plasmapheresis, also known as plasma exchange (PLEX), can be used to induce a remission. This tends to be employed less often today because of the demonstrated efficacy of IVIg and in view of the more invasive nature of PLEX and often the need for admission to the hospital. When PLEX is used successfully, a maintenance dose of corticosteroids is prescribed to decrease the likelihood of relapse. When chronic corticosteroid use is necessary for the treatment of CIDP, it carries significant risk of morbidity. Therefore, many experts prefer to add a variety of other immunosuppressive drugs, as "steroid-sparing agents," to lower the dose of corticosteroids necessary. With the judicious use of individualized therapy, most patients can eventually achieve remission and nearly 80% may make a very good functional improvement.

KEY POINTS TO REMEMBER

- CIDP characteristically involves proximal muscles more than distal and lower limbs more than upper ones. Motor symptoms and signs are more prominent than sensory findings. The course often progresses over many months.

- The diagnosis of CIDP is supported by electrodiagnostic studies, which typically show asymmetric slowing of motor conduction and partial conduction block.
- CSF in CIDP shows the characteristic picture of cyto-albuminologic dissociation.
- Administration of IVIg has become the mainstay of therapy, but plasmapheresis is also effective.

Further Reading

Hughes RA, Donofrio P, Dalakas MC, et al. Intravenous immunoglobulin (10% caprylate-chromatography purified) for the treatment of chronic inflammatory demyelinating polyradiculoneuropathy (ICE study): a randomized placebo-controlled trial. *Lancet Neurol* 2008; 7(2):136-144.

Joint Task Force of the EFNS and the PNS. European Federation of Neurological Societies/Peripheral Nerve Society Guideline on management of chronic inflammatory demyelinating polyradiculoneuropathy: report of a joint task force of the European Federation of Neurological Societies and the Peripheral Nerve Society—First Revision. *J Peripher Nerv Syst* 2010; 15(1):1-9.

Lewis RA. Chronic inflammatory demyelinating polyneuropathy. *Neurol Clin* 2007; 25(1):71-87.

Tracy JA, Dyck PJ. Investigations and treatment of chronic inflammatory demyelinating polyradiculoneuropathy and other inflammatory demyelinating polyneuropathies. *Curr Opin Neurol* 2010; 23(3):242-248.

26 Bickerstaff's Brain Stem Encephalitis

A 53-year-old neurologist presents with two days of double vision and unsteady gait. He describes the double vision as horizontal and present in all directions of gaze, and reports he has been walking "like I am drunk." He denies any associated nausea, vomiting, vertigo, hearing loss, facial numbness or weakness. There is no associated limb weakness, sensory loss, or bowel and bladder dysfunction. His symptoms developed gradually two weeks after a prodromal viral upper respiratory infection. Since then, he has been experiencing a mild headache, malaise, and some confusion and forgetfulness, but denies any fevers or chills. He has been examining his own deep tendon reflexes, which he reports were previously brisk but were difficult to elicit since yesterday. On examination, he is somnolent but easily arousable. His mentation is slow, but he is fully oriented with the exception of the day of the week. Registration is intact, but short-term memory is 2 out of 3 despite prompting. Cranial nerve examination reveals sluggishly reactive pupils and complete ophthalmoplegia in all directions of gaze. Motor and sensory examinations are intact, except for diffuse bilateral hyporeflexia with extensor plantar responses. There is mild to moderate dystaxia with heel-knee-shin testing, and his gait is slightly wide-based with poor tandem walking. General examination is unremarkable without evidence of meningismus. An MRI of the brain demonstrates patchy T2/FLAIR hyperintensities involving the bilateral inferior colliculi with faint enhancement. Lumbar puncture demonstrates a moderate pleocytosis of 23 cells with lymphocytic predominance and an elevated protein level of 75. Serologies for collagen vascular disease, as well as an ACE level, are negative. CSF studies for viruses, Lyme, Whipple's, and *Listeria* are negative. Cytology is also normal. Electromyographic and nerve conduction velocity (EMG/NCV) studies reveal prolonged F-wave responses but are otherwise normal. A GQ1b antibody titer is elevated.

What do you do now?

This patient presents with a post-infectious constellation of findings, including ophthalmoplegia, ataxia, hyporeflexia, and extensor plantar responses, in addition to alteration in consciousness. This presentation of encephalopathy with bulbar, cerebellar, and upper and low motor neuron features localizes the process to the cortex, brain stem and peripheral nervous system. Several infectious and inflammatory conditions should be considered here that can produce a rhomboencephalitis and peripheral neuropathy. The differential diagnosis includes infectious etiologies such as acute botulism, diphtheritic polyneuropathy, Whipple's disease, neuroborrelosis, viral infections such as herpesviridae and HIV, in addition to bacterial infections such as *Listeria* monocytogenes, tuberculosis, and *Mycoplasma pneuomoniae*. In the absence of an acute infectious process, inflammatory or vasculitic etiologies should be considered, such as neurosarcoidosis, Behçet's disease, as well as neoplastic processes such as leptomeningeal carcinomatosis. When the diagnostic evaluation for these entities is unremarkable, an autoimmune process should be considered. The symptomatology involved, specifically the triad of ophthalmoplegia, ataxia, and hyporeflexia, is raises strong clinical suspicion for the Miller Fisher variant of Guillain-Barré syndrome (GBS). This triad, coupled with encephalopathy and the presence of anti-ganglioside antibodies, is pathognomonic for the condition Bickerstaff's brain stem encephalitis (BBE).

BBE is an idiopathic autoimmune disorder that typically presents with acute to progressive cranial nerve dysfunction, usually ophthalmoplegia, associated with cerebellar ataxia, depressed reflexes, and altered mental status, potentially progressing to coma. Bickerstaff first described this disorder in 1957, reporting eight patients with "brainstem encephalitis," who presented with symptoms of drowsiness, acute ophthalmoplegia, ataxia, extensor plantar responses, and hemisensory loss. Whether BBE is considered part of a clinical continuum of anti-ganglioside–mediated neurologic syndromes, such as GBS and its Miller Fisher variant, versus a distinct clinical entity has long been debated and remains controversial. In general, Miller Fisher syndrome can be distinguished clinically from BBE by the absence of upper motor neuron findings and lack of alteration in mental status.

BBE commonly presents in adulthood, but pediatric cases have also been described. Cases are primarily monophasic and remitting with good outcomes, but rare cases of recurrent, relapsing BBE have been reported. In general, the presentation is commonly post-infectious, frequently following a prodromal viral-like illness, and several infections have been implicated, including *Campylobacter jejuni*, cytomegalovirus, typhoid, and *Mycoplasma pneumoniae*. In addition to ophthalmoplegia, commonly presenting bulbar symptoms include facial diplegia and pupillary abnormalities. Flaccid limb weakness has also been described and is considered supportive for an overlapping continuum with the axonal variant of GBS. Deep tendon reflexes can be either hyperreactive or hyporeactive with variable plantar responses.

The presence of anti-GQ1b antibodies and an abnormal brain MRI can help to support the diagnosis of BBE; however, absence of anti-GQ1b antibodies and a normal MRI do not exclude the diagnosis, which remains based on clinical criteria and exclusion of other etiologies that can produce encephalopathy, brain stem syndrome and peripheral nerve dysfunction. A review of 62 patients with BBE identified positive serum anti-GQ1b IgG antibody and MRI brain abnormalities in 66% and 30% of patients, respectively. Brain abnormalities characteristically reveal bilateral brain stem and cerebellar T2/FLAIR hyperintense lesions. CSF studies can demonstrate either an inflammatory signature with lymphocytic pleocytosis or alternatively the characteristic cyto-albuminologic dissociation seen in GBS. EEG studies have also demonstrated abnormalities in patients with altered mental status. Electrophysiologic studies are generally consistent with a peripheral neuropathy involving motor axonal degeneration. Pathologic studies have shown the presence of perivascular lymphocytic infiltration with edema and glial nodules.

The treatment of BBE is generally supportive but can include trials of immunotherapy such as intravenous immunoglobulin or plasma exchange. While the initial presentation is often severe, like GBS, BBE is generally a benign, self-limited illness with good outcome.

KEY POINTS TO REMEMBER

- In BBE, a condition considered possibly related to the Miller Fisher variant of GBS, upper motor neuron features and alteration in consciousness accompany the classic triad of ophthalmoplegia, areflexia, and ataxia.

- Anti-GQ1b antibodies found in Miller Fisher syndrome are also commonly identified in BBE (~66% of cases) and are considered pathogenic.
- The majority of cases of BBE follow a monophasic, remitting course with good outcome, response to immunotherapy such as intravenous immunoglobulin, and rare relapse.

Further Reading

Ito M, Kuwabara S, Odaka M, et al. Bickerstaff's brainstem encephalitis and Fisher syndrome form a continuous spectrum: Clinical analysis of 581 cases. *J Neurol* 2008; 255:674-682.

Odaka M, Yuki N, Yamada M, et al. Bickerstaff's brainstem encephalitis: clinical features of 62 cases and a subgroup associated with Guillain-BarrÈ syndrome. *Brain* 2003; 126:2279-2290.

Overell JR, Willison HJ. Recent developments in Miller Fisher syndrome and related disorders. *Curr Opin Neurol* 2005; 18:562-566.

27 Rassmussen's Encephalitis

A 6-year-old boy presents to his pediatrician with a 2-day
history of left upper and lower limb jerking movements.
The episodes last a few minutes to an hour and resolve
spontaneously. There is no alteration in or loss of
consciousness. His birth and developmental history have
been unremarkable to date. There is no history of head
trauma, meningitis, or stroke. On examination, he is
afebrile with slightly slowed mentation. Funduscopic
examination demonstrates sharp discs without pallor.
Cranial nerves are intact. Motor examination
demonstrates normal tone and slight left pronator drift
with a left-sided reflex preponderance and extensor left
plantar response. Sensory examination is grossly intact
to all modalities. He is admitted to the hospital for
further evaluation for partial motor seizures. A CT of the
head demonstrates right hemispheric atrophy. An MRI of
the brain confirms unihemispheric atrophy without any
discrete lesions or enhancement. Lumbar puncture
demonstrates a mild lymphocytic pleocytosis and
elevated protein, negative bacterial and viral cultures,
and normal cytology. The patient is admitted to the

pediatric intensive care unit. Electroencephalographic monitoring demonstrates background slowing and continuous epileptiform discharges involving the right hemisphere. Antiepileptics are initiated with little clinical improvement.

What do you do now?

Recurrent simple focal clonic motor seizures are otherwise known as epilepsy partialis continua (EPC). EPC can occur in two different clinical scenarios, referred to as Bancaud 1 and 2 types, which denote either a process resulting from a focal structural abnormality or a progressive autoimmune encephalitis known as Rasmussen's encephalitis (RE), respectively. RE was first described in 1958 by Rasmussen and colleagues as a syndrome of focal seizures occurring in the setting of encephalitis. A rare disorder of the CNS, RE is a controversial entity whose pathogenesis remains elusive. It occurs primarily in children under the age of 10, although adult cases have been described. In about 50% of cases an infectious prodromal illness can be identified within the prior six months. Clinically, after the EPC phase, a progressive cognitive decline and hemiplegia can occur, most prominent during the initial year after onset with subsequent residual but static chronic neurologic deficits. Hemiparesis is present in 50% of cases. Depending on which hemisphere is affected, additional deficits such as hemianopia, cortical sensory loss, and dysphasias can occur. Autoimmune and viral etiologies have been entertained. In contrast to pediatric cases, adult forms have demonstrated a more variable course with a more insidious progression of focal neurologic deficits and cognitive decline. Antibodies against glutamate receptor subunits, glutamate receptor 3 (GluR3) and NMDA-type glutamate receptor 2-Epsilon 2, have been identified in some, but not all, cases. Clinically, the presence of these antibodies is not a specific marker of RE, as they have been identified in other types of non-inflammatory epilepsies and have been absent in patients with RE. While several members of the herpesviridae family (Epstein-Barr, cytomegalovirus) also have been implicated, a specific, unifying infectious agent has not been identified.

For unclear reasons, RE tends to be anatomically restricted to a single hemisphere, and neuroimaging reflects a progressive hemispheric atrophy along with focal white matter hyperintensity as well as atrophy of the basal ganglia primarily involving the caudate nucleus head. Pathologic examination of diseased brain tissue demonstrates an inflammatory process with perivascular cuffing of lymphocytes and monocytes involving both gray and white matter, glial nodules, and chronic areas of spongy degeneration and gliosis.

In this case, the absence of a focal structural process, for example tumor, infection, or trauma, and the presence of unihemispheric atrophic changes should raise suspicion for RE. Blood tests generally do not provide any diagnostic insight. A lumbar puncture for CSF analysis should be performed to exclude alternative underlying infectious or neoplastic processes. In RE, the CSF profile is typically normal or nonspecific, although the presence of oligoclonal bands has been reported in a number of cases. Beyond CSF studies, a brain biopsy may be considered if the diagnosis remains unclear and a clinical suspicion for a neoplastic process such as lymphoma remains high; however, risks of biopsy need very careful consideration.

Treatment of RE is based on small anecdotal case reports using trials of high-dose corticosteroids and various immunomodulatory and immuno-suppressive agents with mixed results, but in light of the poor prognosis these should be strongly considered. In addition, intravenous gammaglobulin (IVIg) and plasma exchange have also been reported to produce clinical stabilization. IVIg has demonstrated better efficacy in adult forms compared to pediatric cases. Anticonvulsant therapies appear to have little benefit in controlling seizures. Success in halting the associated EPC has been reported using antiviral therapies such as gancyclovir as well as intraventricular interferon alpha. In cases of refractory EPC secondary to RE, neurosurgical consultation for a hemispherectomy should be considered. Surgical excision of the affected hemisphere appears to be the only option with potential to halt the progression of disease. Risks of this procedure need to be weighed carefully when the dominant hemisphere is involved because of the risks of significant neurologic deficits such as language dysfunction.

KEY POINTS TO REMEMBER

- RE is rare and presents typically with recurrent simple focal motor seizures known as epilepsia partialis continua (EPC).
- During the year following the EPC phase of RE, a progressive cognitive decline and hemiplegia develop; they generally result in residual neurologic deficits.
- The characteristic pathology of RE involves a unihemispheric inflammatory process evolving into corresponding focal atrophy.

- Therapeutic strategies for RE include corticosteroids and immunomodulatory or immunosuppressant regimens, with mixed results.
- The prognosis is poor and in refractory cases unihemispherectomy is considered.

Further Reading

Andrews PI, McNamara JO. Rasmussen's encephalitis: an autoimmune disorder? *Curr Opin Neurobiol* 1996; 6:673-678.

Granata T. Rasmussen's syndrome. *Neurol Sci* 2003; 24:S239-S243.

Hart Y. Rasmussen's encephalitis. *Epileptic Disorders* 2004; 6:133-144.

28 Autoimmune Limbic Encephalitis

A 49-year-old female smoker with a history of depression was brought into the emergency room by ambulance after she had a seizure at home. The event was witnessed by her daughter, who described initial right limb shaking with subsequent loss of consciousness and generalized tonic-clonic movements lasting for approximately 2 minutes. According to her daughter, she has not been herself over the past few weeks, appearing more depressed and forgetful. Her family attributed this to worsening depression, and her psychiatrist increased her sertraline dose last week. The daughter also reports the patient appeared paranoid at times, expressing worry about their water supply being poisoned by chemicals from a nearby factory. In the emergency room, she was postictal with gradual recovery of alertness; however, she was confused and irritable with slowed mentation and poor short-term memory. Further neurologic examination demonstrated mild right upper extremity weakness and bilaterally extensor plantar responses. General examination was unremarkable, without evidence of rashes or meningismus. A non-contrast CT scan of the head and plain chest radiography were normal. An MRI of the brain with and without gadolinium demonstrated enhancing T2/FLAIR hyperintensities bilaterally involving the anteromedial temporal lobes (Figs. 28-1 and 28-2). An electroencephalogram (EEG) showed bilateral slowing with intermittent spikes in the temporal lobes. A lumbar puncture was performed and CSF studies demonstrated 15 white blood cells with a lymphocytic pleocytosis, elevated protein of 76, and normal cytology and flow cytometry. Viral polymerase chain reaction assays, including herpes simplex virus-2 (HSV-2) and human herpes virus 6 (HHV-6), as well as bacterial and fungal cultures, CSF VDRL, 14-3-3 protein, and HIV testing were negative. No toxic/metabolic derangements were identified, including vitamin B12, thyroid function, thiamine levels, and urine and serum toxicology screening. During admission, she had a second partial motor seizure and was loaded with intravenous phenytoin. CSF paraneoplastic antibody panel demonstrated an elevated anti-Hu antibody titer.

What do you do now?

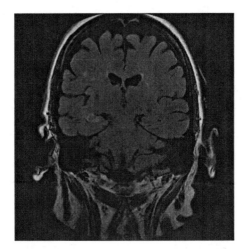

FIGURE 28-1

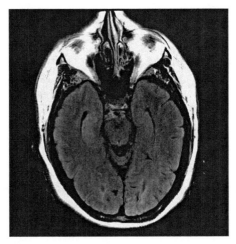

FIGURES 28-1 and 28-2 MRI of the brain (coronal [Fig. 28-1] and axial [Fig. 28-2] FLAIR images) of a 71-year-old woman with a history of confusion, behavioral change, memory impairment, and seizures demonstrating T2/FLAIR hyperintensity involving the right medial temporal lobe, amygdala, and hippocampal regions. Serum voltage-gated potassium channel antibody levels were elevated.

The patient is presenting with an acute to subacute alteration in mental status with neuropsychiatric features and seizures. Infectious causes that should be excluded in this clinical context include CNS viral infections, importantly HSV-2 encephalitis, which has a strong predilection for the anterior temporal lobes, as well as HHV-6, neuroborreliosis, neurosyphilis, and HIV. Noninfectious etiologies to consider include inflammatory conditions such as primary CNS angiitis and lupus cerebritis, neoplastic processes such as lymphomatous meningitis, and toxic/metabolic entities such as Hashimoto's steroid-responsive encephalopathy. Spongiform encephalopathy secondary to prion disease should also be considered in the setting of precipitous cognitive decline and seizures. This patient's MRI, CSF, and EEG findings collectively suggest an inflammatory, noninfectious process targeting the temporal lobes, which is highly suspicious for limbic encephalitis (LE).

Limbic encephalitides are typically autoimmune and often demonstrate protean clinical manifestations. They can be either paraneoplastic or non-paraneoplastic, with a predilection for regions of the medial temporal lobes, such as the hippocampus, amygdala, and orbitofrontal cortices. Lesion development primarily results from a cytotoxic T-cell–mediated inflammatory process. Inflammatory changes involved in autoimmune LE are not, however, restricted to the limbic regions and have been demonstrated in extra-limbic areas, more often than not in the case of paraneoplastic syndromes. Clinically, patients generally present with a rapidly progressive encephalopathy involving memory deficits, seizures, and psychiatric disturbances. The most frequently used diagnostic criteria for paraneoplastic LE are those reported by Gultekin and colleagues, which include the following:

1. Pathologic demonstration of limbic encephalitis, *or*
2. All four of the following:
   a. Symptoms of short-term memory loss, seizures, psychiatric symptoms suggesting involvement of the limbic system
   b. Less than 4 years between the onset of neurologic symptoms and the cancer diagnosis

c. Exclusion of metastasis, infection, metabolic and nutritional deficits, stroke, and side effects of therapy that may cause limbic encephalopathy

d. At least one of the following:
   i. CSF with inflammatory findings
   ii. MRI FLAIR or T2 unilateral or bilateral temporal lobe hyperintensities
   iii. EEG with epileptic or slow activity focally involving the temporal lobes

Determining whether the presenting LE is paraneoplastic or not can pose a significant diagnostic challenge for clinicians, as the neurologic symptoms in 60% to 70% of paraneoplastic cases occur before the identification of the offending tumor, sometimes for years. Several serum and CSF antineuronal autoantibodies directed against onconeural antigens have been described in the setting of LE and can be helpful in narrowing down the differential diagnosis. They are divided into two categories: (1) the classical paraneoplastic intracellular antigens, for example Hu, Yo, CV2/CRMP5, MaTa, and amphiphysin, and (2) cell membrane antigens such as voltage-gated potassium channels (VGKC) and N-methyl-D-asparate (NMDA) receptors, which have been demonstrated in non-paraneoplastic syndromes or in association with atypical tumors, such as thymomas and teratomas. Unfortunately, 40% to 50% of patients with clinical paraneoplastic LE do not possess any of the classic antibodies.

The patient's longstanding history of smoking and positive anti-Hu antibody titer both raise suspicion for an underlying primary lung neoplasm. Therefore, further diagnostic imaging, including a contrast-enhanced CT scan of the chest, abdomen, and pelvis or body [18F]-fluorodeoxyglucose (FDG-PET) scanning, should be performed. While anti-Hu antibody has a strong association with small cell lung cancer, several other antibodies, including anti-CV2/CRMP5, anti-amphiphysin, and anti-Ma, have also been linked to lung neoplasms, both small and non-small cell types, respectively. Of note, anti-Hu antibodies have also been associated with a paraneoplastic sensory polyneuropathy.

Regarding therapeutic options for patients with autoimmune LE, there appear to be two different types of immune-mediated pathophysiology, which correlate with antigen location, and have implications for treatment response. Pathologic studies of LE reveal that those cases associated with intracellular antigens (Hu, CV2/CRMP5, Ma2, amphiphysin) tend to demonstrate a cytotoxic T-cell–mediated inflammatory process, whereas the LE associated with cell membrane antibodies or extracellular antigens (VGKC and NMDA receptors) involves instead an antibody-mediated mechanism with a better response to immunotherapy.

Patients with paraneoplastic autoimmune LE can demonstrate rapid clinical deterioration, and therefore treatment of the underlying malignancy in addition to immunotherapy should be considered. Removal of the neoplasm is sometimes essential for neurologic stabilization or possible improvement. Immunotherapeutic options include courses of intravenous high-dose corticosteroids or intravenous immunoglobulin (IVIg) as well as plasma exchange. More recently, B-cell–targeted therapies such as rituximab have been reported to improve outcomes in patients not responding to the aforementioned therapeutics. Such therapies should be strongly considered early on, even prior to results of autoantibody testing, as affected individuals are sometimes only poorly responsive to treatment.

KEY POINTS TO REMEMBER

- Autoimmune limbic encephalitis can be paraneoplastic or non-paraneoplastic and commonly presents with acute onset of short-term memory loss, confusion, psychiatric features, and seizures.
- The diagnosis of autoimmune LE depends on the clinical picture combined with paraclinical evidence of MRI and EEG abnormalities involving the temporal lobes as well as inflammatory changes in the CSF.
- If a tumor is identified in a patient with a possible paraneoplastic disorder, removal of the tumor has the potential to improve or stabilize neurologic symptoms in some cases.
- Non-paraneoplastic limbic encephalitides may be more common and have a better therapeutic response to immunotherapy.

Further Reading

Graus F, Saiz A, Lai M, et al. Neuronal surface antigen antibodies in limbic encephalitis. *Neurology* 2008; 71:930-936.

Gultekin HS, Rosenfeld MR, Voltz R, Eichen J, Posner JB, Dalmau J. Paraneoplastic limbic encephalitis: neurological symptoms, immunological findings and tumour association in 50 patients. *Brain* 2000; 123:1481-1494.

Tuzun E, Dalmau J. Limbic encephalitis and variants: Classification, diagnosis and treatment. *Neurologist* 2007; 13:261-271.

29 NMDA Receptor Encephalitis

A 25-year-old woman was transferred from a psychiatric hospital after a seizure. Her husband witnessed the event and describes two minutes of whole body shaking accompanied by urinary incontinence and subsequent drowsiness and confusion. Over the past 3 weeks, he reports that she has not been herself, appearing very depressed and anxious and having difficulty remembering things. In addition, he describes she was having bizarre paranoid delusions that her neighbors tapped their telephone line. He also notes that the right side of her face has been intermittently twitching. Two weeks prior, she saw her primary physician for headaches, occasional chills, and cough and was treated for an upper respiratory infection. During that visit, her physician also referred her to a psychiatrist for depression management, and she was prescribed an antidepressant medication, which she never started. The following week she developed suicidal ideations and was admitted for psychiatric hospitalization. On examination, she has a low-grade temperature of 100.2°F and heart rate of 110. Her neck is supple without meningismus.

Upon neurologic examination, she is awake, agitated, easily distractible, and oriented to self only. Her affect is flattened. Speech is pressured but clear and fluent, and she is able to follow simple commands. Cranial nerve examination is grossly normal except for right-sided orofacial dyskinesias. Motor examination demonstrates normal tone and full power throughout with brisk, symmetric deep tendon reflexes and bilaterally extensor plantar responses. Laboratory studies include a normal complete blood count, chemistries, liver function tests, urinalysis, and normal erythrocyte sedimentation rate and TSH and vitamin B12 levels. Serum and urine toxicology are negative. An MRI of the brain with gadolinium contrast is normal. Lumbar puncture demonstrates a lymphocytic pleocytosis with elevated protein and negative encephalitis panel testing for West Nile virus and herpes simplex virus-2 (HSV-2). CSF studies for Lyme and syphilis are negative, and cytology is normal. Continuous electroencephalography (EEG) demonstrates bilateral hemispheric slowing and disorganization. Conventional serum and CSF paraneoplastic autoantibody testing is unremarkable. A contrast-enhanced CT scan of the chest, abdomen, and pelvis searching for an occult tumor, however, reveals a small right-sided ovarian mass suspicious for a teratoma.

What do you do now?

Encephalitis in the setting of an ovarian tumor should raise suspicion for anti-N-methyl-D aspartate-receptor (NMDAR) encephalitis, a recently described paraneoplastic syndrome, which is typically underdiagnosed and can be fatal. Maintaining a high level of clinical suspicion in cases of unexplained encephalitides in young persons, particularly women, is critical, as NMDAR encephalitis is a potentially treatable, reversible condition. The differential diagnosis as expected includes a search for infectious, inflammatory, autoimmune, and paraneoplastic causes of encephalitis, as well as toxic/metabolic encephalopathies.

Characteristic clinical features of NMDAR encephalitis include neuropsychiatric disturbances, including psychosis, decreased levels of consciousness, and memory impairment. There appears to be a characteristic prodromal viral-like illness, which precedes the onset of psychobehavioral symptoms by almost a week. Seizures in addition to bizarre, involuntary choreoathetoid movements of the limbs and orofacial dyskinesias, such as grimacing, masticatory movements, and forceful jaw opening and closing, are common. Patients can demonstrate autonomic instability with cardiac dysrhythmias, labile blood pressure, hyperthermia, and diaphoresis. Central hypoventilation is a characteristic feature in approximately 82% of patients, often requiring long-term mechanical ventilatory support. The majority of patients are initially evaluated by psychiatry, and symptoms are at first attributed to a drug-induced psychosis. Psychiatric symptoms can range from depression and paranoid delusions to frank psychosis with visuo-auditory hallucinations and catatonia. Clinical deterioration can progress to status epilepticus, coma, respiratory failure, and death.

Approximately half of affected patients will demonstrate MRI brain abnormalities affecting various regions, including the medial temporal lobes, cerebral cortex, brain stem, cerebellum, as well as the basal ganglia. Contrast enhancement with gadolinium has been demonstrated in the cerebral cortices, overlying the meninges, and the basal ganglia. The remaining half of patients generally have normal neuroimaging, in concert with pathologic studies that highlight the paucity of inflammatory infiltrates in this disorder. The majority of patients, approximately 90%, will demonstrate both EEG and CSF abnormalities. EEG findings can range from background slowing to status epilepticus. CSF studies typically reveal a mild lymphocytic pleocytosis with elevated protein levels, and oligoclonal bands have been reported.

The pathophysiology of disease appears to involve an antibody-mediated reduction in cell-surface NMDA receptors and clusters of receptors involving postsynaptic dendrites. Autoantibodies in the serum or CSF are directed against the NR1/NR2B heteromer subunits of NMDA-type glutamate receptors localized in postsynaptic membranes, which serve as ligand-gated cation channels that play an important role in synaptic transmission and plasticity. Pharmacologic blockade of these receptors in animals has been shown to produce a clinical picture resembling anti-NMDA receptor encephalitis.

While the majority of cases of NMDAR encephalitis have been reported in the setting of an associated tumor, cases have also appeared that predate identification of the tumor for months to years, as well as in patients without any evidence of occult tumors. Sixty per cent of patients have tumors, which demonstrate the presence of some form of neural tissue. The most common neoplasms associated with this syndrome have been ovarian tumors, primarily teratomas in young women; however, the full clinical spectrum of presentations and treatment responses is not yet clear. Cases associated with teratoma of the testis and small cell lung cancer in male patients have been reported, as well as pediatric cases. NMDA receptor antibodies have also been reported in association with cases of recurrent optic neuritides and seronegative neuromyelitis optica.

Patients with NMDAR encephalitis generally require extensive periods of supportive treatment in intensive care units, often requiring mechanical ventilation. Prompt removal of the offending tumor and immunotherapies to remove autoantibodies have been shown to expedite recovery and even reverse the symptomatology of anti-NMDA receptor encephalitis, although clinical improvement has been described as slow with possible recurrence, particularly if tumor removal and treatment occur late in the course of illness. Cases have been reported to resolve without tumor removal; however, the duration and severity of illness argues strongly in support of therapeutic intervention. Patients who recover have demonstrated a characteristic residual persistent amnesia compatible with disturbance of NMDA receptor-dependent learning and memory. Immunotherapeutic options for NMDAR encephalitis include intravenous high-dose corticosteroids, immunoglobulin and plasmapheresis, as well as cyclophosphamide and rituximab in cases unresponsive to these therapies. Optimal care for patients with anti-NMDA receptor encephalitis should involve a multidisciplinary team approach including coordination among subspecialties of neurology, psychiatry, pediatrics, oncology, and gynecology. The diagnosis should be considered early in cases of encephalitis of unknown origin, new-onset neuropsychiatric disorders, and drug-induced psychosis and in cases of new-onset refractory epilepsy in young persons, particularly women.

KEY POINTS TO REMEMBER

- NMDAR encephalitis is a severe, but often reversible, form of encephalitis associated with autoantibodies to the NR1-NR2 heteromers of the NMDA receptor.
- NMDAR encephalitis predominantly affects young women with ovarian tumors but has also been described in cases without tumors, men, and children.
- The stereotypical clinical course of NMDAR encephalitis involves a viral-like prodrome followed by psychosis, decreased consciousness, hypoventilation, dysautonomia, and dyskinetic movements.
- Prognosis relates to early diagnosis and implementation of immunotherapy and, in paraneoplastic cases, complete tumor removal.

Further Reading

Dalmau J, Gleichman AJ, Hughes EG, et al. Anti-NMDA-receptor encephalitis: case series and analysis of the effects of antibodies. *Lancet Neurol* 2008; 7:1091-1098.

Iizuka T, Sakai F, Ide T, et al. Anti-NMDA receptor encephalitis in Japan: long-term outcome without tumor removal. *Neurology* 2008; 70:504-511.

Irani SR, Bera K, Waters P, et al. N-methyl-D-aspartate antibody encephalitis: temporal progression of clinical and paraclinical observations in a predominantly non-paraneoplastic disorder of both sexes. *Brain* 2010; 133:1655-1667.

Stiff Person Syndrome

A 32-year-old schoolteacher with type 1 diabetes mellitus is referred to a general neurologist for evaluation of six months of back pain and spasms. She reports the pain is difficult to describe in quality but is diffuse, spanning her entire spine and exacerbated by emotional stressors. There is no history of trauma, motor vehicle accidents, or scoliosis. On two occasions, while at work, she experienced a very severe intensifying of the pain, causing her to leave her job early. Her most recent severe episode occurred last week when friends and family threw her a surprise birthday party and upon entering the room she developed very severe shoulder and scapular stiffening after the guests yelled "Surprise!", causing her to leave the party immediately. She is very embarrassed and anxious when relating this experience. Her primary care physician obtained an MRI of the lumbosacral spine, which was normal. A short course of three weeks of physical therapy did not provide any significant benefits and over-the-counter anti-inflammatory medications such as ibuprofen do not seem to help. There is no history of fevers, chills, weight loss, rashes, or adenopathy. Apart from her insulin pump and a low dose of an angiotensin receptor blocker she does not take any medications. Her HbA1c of 6 is in good range, and she denies any significant glycemic abnormalities surrounding these episodes. She reports her relationship with her fiancé is becoming increasingly strained as a result of the pain and anxiety regarding her symptoms and her reluctance to engage in extracurricular activities because of an escalating fear of falling. Over the past few weeks, she reports she has had to move her limbs and back more slowly as quick abrupt movements seem to precipitate attacks. She is referred for neurologic evaluation, and her neurologic examination is entirely normal, although her upright posture appears hyperextended. There is no evidence of motor weakness, spasticity, loss of bulk, or sensory deficits. Her deep tendon reflexes are symmetrically normoactive and plantar responses are bilaterally flexor. Laboratory studies, including complete blood counts, chemistries, liver panel, thyroid function tests, vitamin B12, folate, methylmalonic acid, erythrocyte sedimentation rate, and CPK, are all normal. An MRI of the cervical and thoracic spine is unremarkable. Electromyography with nerve conduction velocity studies demonstrates continuous motor unit activity in agonist and antagonist muscle groups. In light of this finding, an anti-glutamic acid decarboxylase antibody is ordered, and the titer is significantly elevated.

What do you do now?

Chronic back pain is one of the most common complaints of patients presenting for neurologic evaluation. A detailed history and neurologic examination should be performed, seeking evidence for common etiologies such as musculoskeletal strain, degenerative disc disease, and radiculopathy. In the absence of any focal neurologic deficits and a normal MRI of the lumbosacral spine, a conservative approach with a course of physical therapy and over-the-counter anti-inflammatory drugs is reasonable; however, the persistence and severity of this patient's complaint warrant further investigation for alternative, less common, causes. Although she has a clear history of exacerbation from psychosocial stressors, a psychogenic or somatoform etiology should be considered a diagnosis of exclusion after other possible causes are evaluated. For example, paroxysmal events such as tonic spasms secondary to demyelinating disease can also present with recurrent painful spasms secondary to an associated myelopathy; however, these are typically focal, involving one or two limbs, and neurologic examination may demonstrate evidence of myelopathy. Further imaging involving the cervicothoracic spine could be considered in this context. Metabolic derangements such as electrolyte disarray can also be a common cause of painful episodic muscle cramping. In the absence of a structural process or systemic toxic/metabolic derangement, a primary muscle disorder or myopathy could be considered; however, clinically this patient's history and examination do not demonstrate the hallmark proximal muscle weakness typical of a myopathic process. Neuromyotonia, a peripheral nerve disorder, can also produce episodic painful muscle spasms, but these tend to affect primarily the distal musculature.

The electrophysiologic finding of continuous motor activity in agonist and antagonist muscle groups demonstrated by electromyography and nerve conduction velocities is pathognomonic for the condition stiff person syndrome (SPS), previously referred to as stiff man syndrome. SPS, first described in 1956 by Moersch and Woltman, is a rare neuroimmunologic disorder characterized by progressive muscular rigidity, painful spasms primarily involving the axial musculature, and gait impairment due to continuous motor activity. The exact incidence of SPS is unknown, but it tends to affect women more than men and usually presents in the third to sixth decades of life. Symptoms typically begin episodically with an initial fluctuating pattern that subsequently transforms into sustained contractions that limit trunk bending and restrict gait, instilling a fear of falling. Facial stiffness and oculomotor abnormalities ("stiff eyes") have also been described. Symptoms often dissipate during sleep. Paroxysmal autonomic dysfunction has also been reported in cases of SPS, causing episodic diaphoresis, tachycardia, hyperpyrexia, and hypertension with the possibility of sudden death. Seizures have also been reported.

Diagnostic criteria for SPS were proposed in 1989 and include the following:

1. Initial stiffness and rigidity in the axial muscles
2. Slow progression of stiffness to include proximal limb muscles, making volitional movements and ambulation difficult
3. A fixed deformity of the spine, such as lordosis, and with some patients a restriction of hip movement
4. The presence of superimposed episodic spasms precipitated by sudden movements, jarring noise, and emotional upset
5. Normal findings on motor and sensory nerve examinations
6. Normal intellect

While the neurologic examination tends to be normal, exaggerated stretch reflexes and loss of abdominal cutaneous reflexes have been described.

The pathophysiology of SPS remains unknown, but a growing body of evidence favors an autoimmune encephalomyelopathic disorder, possibly antibody-mediated. Autoantibodies against the presynaptic inhibitory epitopes on the enzyme glutamic acid decarboxylase (GAD) and the synaptic membrane protein amphiphysin have been implicated. Anti-GAD antibodies are detected in approximately 60% of cases, but their role in the pathogenesis of SPS remains unclear. In patients seronegative for anti-GAD antibodies, anti-amphiphysin antibodies have been described and appear to have a strong association with underlying malignancy, suggesting a paraneoplastic syndrome. Patients with SPS frequently have comorbid autoimmune diseases, such as type 1 diabetes mellitus, which has been reported in 60% of cases, autoimmune thyroiditis, myasthenia gravis, and pernicious anemia. Several clinical variants of non-paraneoplastic SPS have been described, referred to as SPS-plus syndromes, such as progressive encephalomyelitis with rigidity and myoclonus (PERM) a severe, rapidly progressive disorder with cranial nerve, brain stem, and long tract involvement that distinguishes it from classical SPS.

Because of the rarity of SPS, there are no large-scale controlled clinical trials of therapies. SPS often responds well to medications that increase cortical and spinal inhibition such as the antispasmodic benzodiazepine diazepam. In cases not responsive to diazepam, anti-gamma-aminobutyric acid (GABA) therapy with baclofen, either oral or intrathecal, has been shown to be effective. Corticosteroids have been used in cases refractory to diazepam and baclofen. In addition, various antiepileptic medications have been used, as well as immunotherapies such as corticosteroids, intravenous immunoglobulin, plasmapheresis, and B-cell–depletion therapy with rituximab. Early treatment is critical to prevent long-term development of permanent disability. Injections of botulinum toxin have been reported to produce reduction in hypertonicity, improve ambulation, and decrease pain. Tricyclic antidepressants consistently worsen pain from SPS and should be avoided.

Approximately 5% of SPS cases represent a paraneoplastic syndrome; therefore, whole body CT scan imaging for an occult malignancy should be strongly considered. The most common associated malignancies are breast and small cell lung cancer. If an occult malignancy is identified, treatment of the tumor or neoplastic process can sometimes, but not always, results in improvement in the associated paraneoplastic phenomenon.

As SPS progresses, patients often require ambulatory assistive devices. Care should be taken to avoid the possibility of limb fractures secondary to loss of postural reflexes in the setting of hypertonia and superimposed severe spasms. Emotional and psychosocial support should be provided, as patients frequently demonstrate comorbid anxiety and depressive disorders either in conjunction with or secondary to the emotional stress of the symptoms.

KEY POINTS TO REMEMBER

- SPS is characterized by progressive muscle rigidity and stiffness accompanied by painful spasms of the axial musculature and gait impairment associated with the presence of elevated titers of anti-GAD antibodies.
- Electromyography in SPS demonstrates the typical pattern of continuous low-frequency firing of normal motor units simultaneously in both agonist and antagonist muscle groups.

- In patients with a strong clinical suspicion for SPS who are seronegative for anti-GAD antibody, anti-amphiphysin antibodies should be tested to evaluate for the possibility of an associated paraneoplastic syndrome with occult malignancy.

Further Reading

Egwuonwu S, Chedebeau F. Stiff person syndrome: a case report and review of the literature. *J Natl Med Assoc* 2010; 102:1261-1263.

Espay AJ, Chen R. Rigidity and spasms from autoimmune encephalomyelopathies: stiff-person syndrome. *Muscle Nerve* 2006; 34:677-690.

Murinson BB. Stiff-person syndrome. *Neurologist* 2004; 10:131-137.

Index